Clinician's Guide to

Spirituality

Notice

Medicine is an ever-changing science. As new research and clinical experience broaden our knowledge, changes in treatment and drug therapy are required. The authors and the publisher of this work have checked with sources believed to be reliable in their efforts to provide information that is complete and generally in accord with the standards accepted at the time of publication. However, in view of the possibility of human error or changes in medical sciences, neither the authors nor the publisher nor any other party who has been involved in the preparation or publication of this work warrants that the information contained herein is in every respect accurate or complete, and they disclaim all responsibility for any errors or omissions or for the results obtained from use of the information contained in this work. Readers are encouraged to confirm the information contained herein with other sources. For example and in particular, readers are advised to check the product information sheet included in the package of each drug they plan to administer to be certain that the information contained in this work is accurate and that changes have not been made in the recommended dose or in the contraindications for administration. This recommendation is of particular importance in connection with new or infrequently used drugs.

Clinician's Guide to
Spirituality

Bowen F. White, M.D.

Founding Member, American Holistic Medical Association
Founding Member, American Board of Holistic Medicine
Adjunct Clinical Assistant Professor
Department of Preventive Medicine
University of Kansas School of Medicine
Corporate Medical Consultant, Hazelden Foundation

John A. Mac Dougall, D.Min.

Supervisor of Spiritual Care, Hazelden Foundation
Associate Professor of Chemical Dependency Counseling
Hazelden Graduate School of Addiction Studies
Clinical Member, Association for Clinical Pastoral Education

McGraw-Hill
Medical Publishing Division

New York   Chicago   San Francisco   Lisbon   London   Madrid   Mexico City
Milan   New Delhi   San Juan   Seoul   Singapore   Sydney   Toronto

9/2001

McGraw-Hill

*A Division of The **McGraw·Hill** Companies*

1 2 3 4 5 6 7 8 9 0 DOC DOC 0 9 8 7 6 5 4 3 2 1

ISBN 0-07-134717-8

This book was set in Korinna by Keyword Publishing Services.
The editor was Martin Wonsiewicz.
The production supervisor was Catherine Saggese.
Project management was provided by Keyword Publishing Services.
The cover design was by Aimee Nordin.
R.R. Donnelley & Sons was the printer and binder.

This book is printed on acid-free paper.

Library of Congress Cataloging-in-Publication Data
White, Bowen Faville, 1946–
    Clinician's guide to spirituality / authors, Bowen F. White, John A. Mac Dougall.
        p.; cm.
    Includes bibliographical references and index.
    ISBN 0-07-134717-8
        1. Medical care—Religious aspects.   2. Medical care—Moral and ethical aspects.
    3. Patients—Religious life.   4. Spiritual healing.   5. Spirituality—Health aspects.
    I. Mac Dougall, John A., D.Min.   II. Title.
        [DNLM: 1. Physicians—psychology.   2. Religion and Medicine.   3. Ethics, Medical.
    4. Physician–Patient Relations.   W50 W582c 2001]
    R725.55.W48 2001
    291.1'78321—dc21   00-050099

To all my patients who have honored me by letting me doctor them and, as a result, have become my teachers on the spiritual path.

B.F.W.

To my wife, Priscilla; my daughters, Priscilla and Chris; and to my good friends Barbara and Sara, who helped me stay alive when the outcome was in doubt.

J.A.M

Contents

PART III. CONCLUSION

Preface

This book explores the impact of spiritual health on the physical, mental, and emotional health of patients and clients. The interplay among these components defines our state of health and well-being in general. Spiritual health means living according to spiritual principles and thereby enhancing our relationships with a Higher Power, with ourselves, and with others. This book is written from two perspectives: a medical doctor (Bowen White) and a chaplain (myself). It is written to inspire you, as clinicians, to attend first to your own spiritual health. We believe we can be more effective caregivers by practicing these principles in our lives. To promote the spiritual health of our patients and clients, we propose sharing these principles and our personal experience, strength, and hope with our patients and clients. Finally, we propose applying these principles in our clinical practices.

■ PUTTING SPIRITUAL PRINCIPLES INTO PRACTICE

Johann Noordsij, M.D., my thesis advisor in my Doctor of Ministry program, was a psychiatrist who specialized in treating severely mentally ill people who were also chemically dependent. I asked him how he knew when his patients were well. He said, "When they can tell their psychiatrist to go fly a kite." I asked if that meant when they were angry with him. He responded, "No, when they can say to me 'Dr. Noordsij, I'm not going to do that, because that's not who I am.' Then they know who they are." I asked how he taught them to be who they are. He said, "I don't. But they learn to be who they are by watching me be who I am." Our patients are watching us be who we are. By attending to our own spirituality, and putting spiritual principles into practice, we can influence who they become and help them lead healthier lives.

The origins of my thoughts about spirituality come from the Twelve Step programs created for the treatment of people with alcoholism and addiction, and for the help of their family members and friends.

■ THE FOUNDATION: SPIRITUALITY

Observations and opinions in this book reflect my professional training and life experiences as a recovering alcoholic and drug addict, a chronic migraine pain patient, and a spiritual care provider in a residential treatment center at Hazelden located in Center City, Minnesota. At Hazelden, the spiritual principles outlined here are used in treating patients with chemical dependency and related issues. These are the principles that form the foundation of the Twelve Steps of Alcoholics Anonymous.

■ TREATING OTHERS WITH DIGNITY AND RESPECT

If we want to improve our spirituality, today, reliably, all we need to do is to treat other human beings as if they were beloved children of their Higher Power. We don't have to personally love them. In some cases, that might be a stretch. But at least imagine that they have a Higher Power, it isn't us, and that their Higher Power loves them. As we start to re-imagine people as children of God, we will begin to treat them with dignity and respect because of our new beliefs. As we do this, our relationships with them will improve because we are respecting their dignity, we'll feel better about ourselves because our conduct is more honorable, and it will gradually dawn on us that if they have a loving Higher Power, so do we. Our whole attitude and outlook on life will change.

■ ESTABLISHING POSITIVE DOCTOR–PATIENT RELATIONSHIPS

How patients and clients are visualized by us will determine the nature of the doctor–patient relationship. In spiritual care, the bright, motivated, honest patient is more fun to be with than the one who is filled with excuses, blame, and denial. If I base my relationship on how much I am enjoying our visit, I will be helpful only to those people whom I like. I might have the same insights for both groups, but how I feel about them will be detected. The unmotivated patient will feel my dislike, and translate it defensively into dislike of me. With the relationship ruined, they are unlikely to benefit from my help. If I look at the patient as a child of God, and a suffering alcoholic and addict, I won't blame them for showing the symptoms of their disease. They will detect my compassionate spirit, and open up.

In the early 1980s I was an ambulance supervisor and worked with the emergency room of a major teaching hospital. They initiated a self-study to determine problem areas. The Emergency Department personnel admitted that they weren't treating drunks well. The ambulance crew's point of view was that, if we brought them in, there was more than drunkenness going on. The medical staff saw these patients as undesirable. They were often unclean, uncooperative, and without money. Triage was minimal, and they were often left in chairs until they went away. Emergency room staff treated the patients they felt were more deserving, not the most seriously ill. The hospital brought in a new emergency room director, who corrected the situation, but this type of triage by attractiveness probably continues in many places, although in more subtle ways.

■ IDENTIFYING A COMMON HUMANITY

My first Clinical Pastoral Education experience was in a large urban hospital. One day I was in an elevator with a group of doctors. They were discussing anatomical parts, not people, "How's the hip you had this morning?" and "I had three heart attacks." I wondered if these hips were attached to people, or if the three heart attacks had happened to three people who had lives outside the emergency room.

Anonymity has very little to do with not using last names in Twelve Step programs, or protecting patients' personal information. That's privacy. Privacy is part of anonymity, but anonymity ultimately has to do with fellowship and equality. It means that we are not identified by our differences, but by our common humanity. We have differences, some of them obvious, but they do not matter very much. We recover in fellowship with other people, not in opposition to them. We give all people the same high value we give ourselves.

■ A CLOSE CALL

Thinking about other people helps us get through difficult situations. In October 1996 my wife and I were going to Thailand on vacation. We had nice first-class seats on the upper deck of Northwest flight 19 from Minneapolis to Tokyo, Japan. The 747-200 aircraft was fully loaded with passengers, luggage, cargo, and fuel. Just as we got off the ground, the right inboard engine disintegrated with a big bang and flames. We wobbled across the Lake Nokomis golf course at treetop level, scaring the golfers. Gradually we gained some height. However, we couldn't land again because the plane was too heavy. It would just smash the landing gear to bits. We flew to Fargo, turned north, dumped 200,000 pounds of jet fuel over the Red River Valley, and looped back toward Minneapolis. The controllers closed the airport, sending all the other planes toward Milwaukee and Duluth. The fire trucks arrived along with the local TV reporters who came to film this disaster in the making. We landed just fine.

On arrival, the majority of the passengers were really ugly about this. Initially they were angry because they had been frightened. Once we were on the ground, they got over being frightened and then became angry when they realized we wouldn't be going to Tokyo today. By the time you go to Los Angeles or San Francisco and change planes, it's a day later because the earth is a sphere. The people with the ugliest dispositions got on television to denounce the airline.

I went up to the pilot and said, "Nice flying. Any landing you walk away from is a good one!" I wasn't thinking, "Me, my will, my life, my vacation, how can Northwest Airlines do this to me!," as if the board of directors had sat around and said, "John's going on vacation, let's blow up a plane." It wasn't about me at all. Spiritual maturity means realizing that not every story is about me. What about the flight crew? This is what they trained for. This is when maturity and experience counts, so congratulations! Sure we got bussed to Edina, Minnesota, instead of flying to Bangkok, but we got there eventually. More importantly, the remainder of my vacation wasn't ruined by resentment about losing the first day. I was able to live in fellowship with the flight crew and fellow passengers, instead of struggling against them in the vain hope of improving my trip. As we grow spiritually, our relationships with the Higher Power, ourselves, and others become more important than getting our way in the present. We lighten up.

John A. Mac Dougall, D.Min.

Preface

As a holistic medical doctor, I view human beings as multidimensional—more than mere physical atoms in a bag of skin that metabolize their way into oblivion. The physical, emotional, mental, and spiritual dimensions are all intertwined. The first three dimensions, connected in psychophysiologic ways as the mind–body connection, allow us to stay within the comfortable realm of science while spirituality is a mysterious dimension that is easier to ignore. Our medical training neglected it because spirituality was viewed as someone else's job: chaplains, counselors, social workers.

My premise is that any health problem may provide an opportunity for learning and personal growth. We can find meaning in any form of suffering, any problem that we experience. My intent here is not to present definitive answers but to provide clues and insights to guide you in a more holistic approach to medical care—to show you my approach, not tell you how to do yours. I invite you to take a glimpse into a domain that reflects my personal biases, and I encourage you to take what is useful and forget the rest.

This book is about taking a journey with suffering people. It represents an inclusive, nondenominational approach to consider as you travel inward with your patients. We all have beliefs that impact how we think, feel, behave, and physically function. Exploring these beliefs is part of treating the whole person.

Bowen F. White, M.D.

Acknowledgments

Thanks to the University of Kansas Medical School for giving me a chance. Thanks also to the good folks at Goppert Family Care Center for understanding my interest in holistic medicine. Thank you Jack S., Jack H., Larry R., Katie, and all the nurses. Thanks also to Coleman Barks and Robert Bly. Thanks to all my mentors living and dead, including the ones I have never met like Rumi who have spoken to me of the friend as a friend.

Thank you to Corrine Casanova for her lightness and buoyancy in approaching this project. Heavy and serious subjects need some balancing energy to keep the words from falling off the page. Likewise my co-author, John Mac Dougall, carries this quality of energy and is a delight and inspiration to others including myself. Thank you, John. Finally, thanks to Hazelden and McGraw-Hill for publishing this work.

B.F.W.

I wish to thank my editor, Corrine Casanova, my co-author, Bowen White, Hazelden Information and Educational Services, and McGraw-Hill for their help in turning this manuscript into a book, and I thank the reader for considering what we have written.

J.A.M.

Clinician's Guide to
Spirituality

I

Part I

Spirituality and Medicine

1

Chapter One

The Research Behind Spirituality and Positive Health Outcomes

John A. Mac Dougall

While a reasonable amount of research has been done on links between spirituality and positive health outcomes, much of this is on religion, rather than spirituality. We define spirituality as the quality or nature of our relationships in three dimensions: with a Higher Power, with ourselves, and with other people. We define religion as a system of beliefs and behaviors that are intended to improve spirituality.

Religion is much more observable than spirituality. Researchers can study church attendance or membership, patterns of beliefs, and specific behavior, such as scripture reading, worship, prayer, and ritual. Spirituality is less easily observed. Our key terms are difficult to quantify: honesty, hope, faith, courage, integrity, willingness, humility, compassion, justice, perseverance, spiritual awareness, and service. It would be difficult to design the traditional double blind test with control groups for research in spirituality. If, for example, we asked one group to be honest, and another to be dishonest, how could we tell if they were being honest about their dishonesty? If we divided seriously ill patients into groups and asked one group to increase their spiritual awareness through prayer and meditation, and asked the other group not to pray, how would we verify that this group of equally sick people were not praying?

Nonetheless, the research that exists indicates that something positive is happening in the link between religion and health. Our suspicion is that spirituality is the active ingredient that makes religion a positive force. Religion can be a passive system of beliefs. Spirituality calls for active involvement in relationships with a higher power, self, and others. It is our relationships, much more than our beliefs, that make us well. This is clear in the realm of physical medicine. Many women believe that mammograms are useful in early detection and treatment of breast cancer, but only those women who form a relationship with the health care system and actually get mammograms will have a positive health outcome. Many smokers believe that smoking is making them sick, and that they would be much better off without smoking, but only those who change their relationship with nicotine will have a positive health outcome. Beliefs may be necessary precursors of spiritual change, but they do not bring about that change alone.

In this chapter, we take a look at representative studies on the impact of religion on health. Elements of religion that have received substantial study include church attendance, religiously based behavior change, and prayer.

Church Attendance and Health

There is a positive correlation between church attendance and positive health care outcome. One early large study covered 91,909 people in Washington County, Maryland who attended church at least weekly. The study found a 53 percent lower death rate from suicide than non-church attendees, 56 percent lower from emphysema, 50 percent lower from coronary artery disease, and 74 percent lower from cirrhosis of the liver. The large number of participants suggests validity, but the study did not control for behavioral factors. It did not tell whether the 56 percent reduction in death from emphysema was because church attendance provided some protection from the dangers of smoking, or whether people who attended church were less likely to smoke at all.[1]

In a California study of 5,286 people from 1965 to 1994, those who attended church regularly had a 36 percent lower chance of dying during the study than the people who attended less than once a week. After discounting for greater social ties and better health practices, the remaining difference was still 23 percent. Women had greater benefit than men. This may relate to the tendency of women to use religion to solve life problems more than men.[2]

Church attendance has a correlation with better immune system function. In a study of 1,718 subjects over age 65, low church attendance was associated with higher levels of interleukin-6 (IL-6) a blood protein that indicates immune system dysfunction. Frequent church attendees were only half as likely to as non-attendees to have high levels of IL-6 in their blood. This suggests stronger immune system function.[3]

Religiously Based Behavior Change and Health

Some religions expect their adherents to make behavior changes to live appropriately. Some of these changes, made for religious reasons, are also related to health.

Mormons have some of the clearest links between religiously dictated behavior and behaviors believed to promote health. Mormons are expected to abstain from alcohol, tobacco, coffee, and tea, and a great many of them do. Other expectations, with less of a physical link to health, are also present: church attendance and living a morally correct life.

Separate studies of Mormon men[4] and women[5] indicated that Mormon men who adhered to the religion well enough to achieve higher priesthood levels were less likely to develop cancer, and the Mormon women who were more involved in their church were less likely to get cancer than those who were less committed to their church. In these cases, the behavior changes required of Mormons may well be added to the less well understood positive effects of faith.

Prayer and Health

In a Duke University study of 3,963 men and women over age 65, researchers followed the surviving members of the group for six years. Factors of age, race, schooling, religious activity and denomination, overall physical health, history of cigarette smoking, body-mass index, and blood pressure were considered. Subjects were asked how often they attended religious services, how frequently they prayed, or studied the Bible. Once all the variables were taken into account, both men and women who both attended religious services and prayed or studied the Bible frequently were 40 percent less likely to have diastolic hypertension than those who did so infrequently.[6]

Not only does the patient's prayer seem to improve health, prayer by others on behalf of the patient seems to have a positive effect, as well. A 1988 study at San Francisco General Hospital studied the effects of intercessory prayer on two groups of coronary care unit patients. The study group of 192 patients received intercessory prayer by people around the country, and a group of 201 patients did not receive such prayer. All knew they were in a study of prayer, but none knew which group they were in. While 27 percent of the patients in the control group had complications, only 15 percent of those being prayed for had complications.[7] This may not have been a perfect double blind study since we cannot know who else was praying, and to what effect, for the patients in the control group. However, any additional prayers for the control group would likely have made the resulting difference less dramatic, instead of exaggerating it.

Spiritual Awareness and Health

There is a positive correlation between a good relationship between the patient and their Higher Power and good health care outcomes. In a 1995 study at Dartmouth Medical School, 232 older patients were followed for six months after the completion of heart surgery. Those who attended church regularly had only about half of the death rate of those who didn't. However, the 37 patients who stated that they derived "strength and comfort" from their beliefs all survived that six month period.[8]

A study of elderly poor people in Connecticut measured "religiousness" which included church attendance, degree of faith, and habits of seeking emotional strength from religion. The non-religious elderly were two and a half times more likely to die during the two-year study period. The researchers isolated the practice of deriving strength from religion as the strongest factor.[9]

In a synthesis of a variety of studies, Dale Matthews, David Larson, and Constance Barry found that religious factors have a positive influence on health. The religious factors vary by study, but 109 of the 131 studies cited showed positive outcomes, for health issues ranging from depression and chemical use to blood pressure and overall survival.[10]

What Doesn't Work

Faith and magic are opposites. In faith, we try to align ourselves to do God's will. In magic, we try to bend God to our will. Some who look at literature on spirituality and health will be looking for magic: the right behavior, the right prayer, the right ritual, to bring about the healing we want. Magical thinking doesn't bring about healing. This is most apparent in the tragic stories of parents withholding treatment from dangerously ill children, in the belief that God will provide a miraculous healing. The belief may appear to be in God, but actually it is in magic. If they believed in a God who could and would heal, and who was much more powerful than people, they would not instruct God to heal using only those means they have chosen. When they say, based on their own will, that God will not use physicians and medicine, then they are acting as God's overseer. They are more committed to having a miracle on their terms than they are to the actual healing. Such cases often end up in court when it becomes apparent that the parents are willing to have their children die rather than abandon their magical belief systems.

Religion that is merely the projection of the religious person's anger is not healthy. All manner of violence and strife over the centuries have been caused or justified by religious belief systems. Religion whose content is based on God's war against one's enemies brings the stress of eternal conflict.

Religion that is based in fear promotes anxiety, not health. Some people who have been taught that their slightest sin causes them to be separated from God and placed in danger of hell. When they are old enough to question whether God is really that angry with them, they often leave that religion in a flight towards health.

How Religion and Spirituality Promote Health

Statistical studies can suggest that there is a causal relationship between church attendance, prayer, and spiritual awareness and good health, but they have not isolated the "active ingredients." Ours is not the only attempt to do so. Dale A. Matthews, M.D., and Connie Clark suggest twelve remedies that draw on spiritual and religious strengths:

1. Equanimity—Overcoming the Wear and Tear of Life
2. Temperance—Honoring the Body as a Temple of the Spirit
3. Beauty—Appreciating Art and Nature
4. Adoration—Worshiping with Our Whole Beings
5. Renewal—Confessing and Starting Over
6. Community—Bearing One Another's Burdens
7. Unity—Getting Strength Through Shared Beliefs
8. Ritual—Taking Comfort in Familiar Activities
9. Meaning—Finding a Purpose in Life
10. Trust—"Letting Go and Letting God"
11. Transcendence—Connecting with Ultimate Hope
12. Love—Caring and Being Cared For [11]

Herbert Benson, M.D., suggests that religious ritual, fellowship, altruism, intercessory prayer, and therapeutic touch are the active ingredients.[12] The twelve factors of honesty, hope, faith, courage, integrity, willingness, humility, compassion, justice, perseverance, spiritual awareness, and service come from the experience of people helping each other in the Twelve Step Programs. These programs were originally developed to treat alcoholism, and are now applied to a variety of addictive diseases and related conditions, with considerable success.

A Higher Power by any name; a plan of spiritual progress and personal responsibility of any kind; faith, hope, love, trust, and comfort in any form; are all likely to promote healing and health. Our book is about one such plan.

REFERENCES

1. G.W. Comstock and K.B. Partridge, "Church Attendance and Health," *Journal of Chronic Diseases* 25 (1972) 665–672.
2. W.J. Strawbridge, et al., "Frequent Attendance at Religious Services and Mortality Over 28 Years," *American Journal of Public Health* 87, no. 6 (June 1997) 957–961.
3. H.G. Koenig, H.J. Cohen, L.K. George, J.C. Hayes, D.B. Larson, and D.G. Blazer "Attendance at Religious Services, Interleukin-6, and Other Biological Indicators of Immune Function In Older Adults," *International Journal of Psychiatry in Medicine* 27 (1997) 233–250.
4. J.W. Gardiner and J.L. Lyon, "Cancer in Mormon Men by Lay Priesthood Level," *American Journal of Epidemiology* 116 (1982) 243–257.
5. J.W. Gardiner and J.L. Lyon, "Cancer in Utah Mormon Women by Church Activity Level," *American Journal of Epidemiology* 116 (1982) 258–264.
6. H.G. Koenig, L.K. George, H.J. Cohen, J.C. Hayes, D.G. Blazer, and D.B. Larson, "The Relationship Between Religious Activities and Blood Pressure in Older Adults," *International Journal of Psychiatry in Medicine* 28 (1998) 189–213.

7. R.B. Byrd, "Positive Therapeutic Effects of Intercessory Prayer in a Coronary Care Unit Population," *Southern Medical Journal* 81 (1988) 826–829.

8. T.E. Oxman, D.H. Freeman, and E.D. Manheimer, "Lack of Social Participation or Religious Strength and Comfort as Risk Factors for Death after Cardiac Surgery in the Elderly," *Psychosomatic Medicine* 57 (1995) 5–15.

9. D.M. Zuckerman, S.V. Kasl, and A.M. Ostfeld, "Psychosocial Predictors of Mortality Among the Elderly Poor," *American Journal of Epidemiology* 119 (1984) 410–423.

10. D.A. Matthews, D.B. Larson, and C.P. Barry, *The Faith Factor: An Annotated Bibliography of Clinical Research on Spiritual Subjects, Vol. 1*, John Templeton Foundation, 1994.

11. D.A. Matthews and C. Clark, *The Faith Factor, Proof of the Healing Power of Prayer*, Penguin Books, New York, 1998, pp. 42–52.

12. H. Benson, *Timeless Healing*, Scribner, New York, 1996, pp. 177–183.

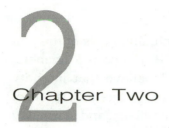

Chapter Two

Spirituality and the Twelve Steps

John A. Mac Dougall

> The spiritual perfection of man consists in his becoming an intelligent being—one who knows all that he is capable of learning.
>
> Maimonides, *The Guide for the Perplexed*, 1190 A.D.

■ DETERIORATING PHYSICIAN–PATIENT RELATIONSHIPS

The public's dissatisfaction with modern medicine is partly due to the weakening of the physician–patient relationship. Under the pressure of managed care, people are sometimes forced to change physicians. Those physicians who are contracted with managed care organizations may be pressured to spend less time with their patients.

As traditional physician–patient relationships wither, the results are as poor for physicians as patients. A Gallup Poll for CNN, broadcast on July 16, 1999, asked about public confidence in institutions. Sixty-eight percent of respondents had confidence in the military, 40 percent in the medical system, and 17 percent in HMOs. What was once a relationship of trust is increasingly

---

The Twelve Steps are reprinted from the Alcoholics Anonymous (A.A.) "Big Book" with permission from Alcoholics Anonymous World Services, Inc.

becoming an adversarial relationship. Ironically, news of the poll was followed by an advertisement for J.P. Morgan, a financial powerhouse, in which the actor stated "I believe that integrity doesn't hinder performance. It is performance." Integrity is one of the spiritual principles recommended for clinicians, and ultimately for patients.

■ POPULARITY OF ALTERNATIVE MEDICINES

The absence of spirituality from modern medicine is a factor in the trend towards alternative medicines, which are viewed as more spiritual than traditional medical care. In 1997, more people visited an alternative therapist than a primary care physician, and Americans spend more than $4 billion on herbal remedies.[1]

Although many alternative therapies range from whimsical to harmful, the relationships between patients and providers are stronger in alternative medicine than in traditional practices. Relationships and spirituality are competing successfully with modern medicine in the marketplace. Patients are choosing enhanced human contact over science. Clinicians can give their patients and clients the best possible care by applying the spiritual principles described in this book along with the best science they, as clinicians, can offer.

Chemical dependency, one of many chronic illnesses, is a useful model for treatment and recovery from chronic illness because it includes all the elements that may be present in other chronic illnesses—including spiritual, emotional, mental, and physical disorders. Many chronic illness patients can limit their disorder to only physical illness, and remain lucid, emotionally appropriate, and spiritually fit. This is unlikely to happen by chance. A process of character development to limit the effects of chronic illness to physical problems, and often to adapt to and reduce those problems is needed, as well. By applying the principles, the patient can be emotionally, physically, and spiritually well. The Twelve Steps that were developed for the treatment of alcoholism have broad application for any chronic illness.

■ SPIRITUAL GROWTH AND RENEWAL

The men and women who developed Alcoholics Anonymous (A.A.) discovered that when they tried to stop drinking, they could quit, but not abstain permanently. When they focused on a program of spiritual growth and renewal, they were able to stay sober. Very little in the Twelve Step programs is actually about "not drinking" or "not taking drugs." The programs are about developing a manner of spiritually healthy living. While developing our spirituality, the burdens of life are eased. While their chronic illnesses aren't gone, they no longer interfere with a good life. For each of the proposed principles, links will be drawn between practicing the principle and having a good life (defined by the patient), even while chronically ill.

■ SPIRIT STRENGTHENING

The universal spiritual principles developed for the relief of alcoholism take hold of alcoholics by strengthening the spirit of their lives. With the development or restoration of spiritual health, the formerly impossible task of living sober becomes simple. The principal task of recovery from addiction develops a way of life in which life is lived on life's terms: a commitment to meet the day's unknown challenges by relying on spirituality and a network of healthy relationships rather than on chemicals. Similarly, the development or restoration of spiritual health gives them strength, comfort, and resilience to face the challenges of any chronic illness, or indeed of life itself. Spiritual health is not necessarily a cure for illness, but it is a fine form of care, making life good even while challenged by an illness or injury. The illness or injury can give a reason for seeking spiritual growth, and thus be a life asset in their lives. Chronic illness can cause them to examine their lives, principles, and values. Physical illness can be the origin of a movement towards spiritual health. Changing their spirituality is a powerful healing tool. It's also a good starting point for clinicians to consider what spirituality is, for themselves, their patients, and the relationships between them.

■ HIGHER POWER, SELF, AND OTHERS

A person's spirituality consists of the quality and nature of their relationships with a Higher Power, with themselves, and others. Whole lives are lived in the context of those three relationships. It isn't possible to separate them by very much. They cannot love God, be at peace with themselves, and treat everybody else like dirt. It just doesn't work out. The moral instruction to "Love your neighbor as yourself" may be taken as religious teaching, but it is also a description of reality. They cannot help loving one's neighbor as oneself. When they regard others with bitterness, it reflects their own bitterness. When they care deeply for others, it shows that they also love themselves and they are connected to the care of a Higher Power.

Any improvement in any one of their relationships with their Higher Power, themselves, or with other people lifts the others. Any deterioration in one of these pulls the other two down. If they go home and have a knock-down drag-out fight with the people they allegedly love, and dig deep for every nasty thing they can say to them to win the fight, by the end of the evening, their relationships will be damaged. In addition, they won't be likely to go to bed and say their prayers, because they'll be embarrassed to talk to God because they've been so tacky. They'll also feel badly about themselves because they will eventually regret what they said. All three relationships will be damaged—Higher Power, self, and others—even though they've only been fighting with others.

■ ANONYMITY

In the Twelve Step programs, the Twelve Steps are for individual conduct and the Twelve Traditions are for group life. By extension, the Traditions can be used for all social relationships. The Twelfth Tradition states that "Anonymity is the spiritual foundation of all our traditions, ever reminding us to place principles above personalities." This tradition, when practiced, enhances spirituality by changing how other people are viewed. Instead of seeing people as diagnoses or pathologies, they are seen as whole.

■ SURPASSING THE MEDICAL HIERARCHY

The medical system is not based on fellowship, but on hierarchy. This may be a necessity of the system as it exists because some-one has to ultimately be in charge. However, it is important for clin-icians to disbelieve in their own importance. Relationships are better served by fellowship and equality than by status conscious-ness. A physician who manages a heart transplant unit recently revealed the ingredients of his happy marriage by stating, "It's very simple. I'm a god at work. I'm not a god at home."

■ RATING OTHERS

A normal but unhealthy way for people to relate to others is to grade them, according to how well they are pleasing them right now. For example, if they are looking for potential dates, their grades will be the algebraic functions of attractiveness times avail-ability. If they are looking for advancement on the job, other peo-ple's grades will be based on the statistical probability that they will network with them, directly or indirectly, to get them the jobs of their dreams. If they are seeking power or prestige, other peo-ple's grades will be the sum of their behaviors that make them look good. This could be either by flattering them, or by providing a pitiful example or well-timed failure with which they could con-trast themselves. In all cases, their grades are based on others, not on them. Their evaluation of their value is based on what they want, not on who they are.

In the application of the spiritual principle of anonymity, they give up the whole grading business. They no longer act as if they are the center of the universe, and they recognize the validity and value of other people's lives. They gradually lose their self-centeredness, and assume that other people's lives matter as much as theirs does. As they apply this principle, they develop a more spiritual response to all kinds of situations.

■ THE CHALLENGE OF THE CHRONICALLY ILL PATIENT

Clinicians are more comfortable with people who recover because they make the clinicians feel successful. Clinicians naturally prefer the acutely ill because they are likely to make dramatic progress and in turn validate the clinicians' skills. Chronically ill patients tend to be less desired, in part because they are not as likely to experience dramatic improvement and thus make the clinician feel good. When practicing the principle of anonymity, the patients' experience of cure, care, and comfort becomes more important than the clinician's own needs for success. It becomes more important that the patients get help than it is that the clinicians be viewed as helpers.

Religion and Spirituality

■ IN THE FACE OF CHRONIC ILLNESS

Chronic illness presents the patient and the physician with the limits of their powers. Commonly, chronic illness cannot be made to go away. A positive outcome is that it is successfully managed, not gone. Patients faced with their own limited power naturally turn to either an ultimate power or principles of ultimate value. When they cannot solve a problem, they look to solutions beyond themselves. The alternative is to get stuck in resentment and self pity.

The chronic illness patient can either turn to religion for the assurance of a Higher Power's ultimate care, turn to spiritual principles to improve the quality of life, or turn inward and withdraw from life. Ideally, they can avoid the withdrawal and use both spirituality and religion.

Religions are systems of beliefs and behaviors that are intended to improve spirituality. They may or may not, depending on the quality and nature of the relationships within the religion.

■ THE KILLER NUN STORY

In chemical dependency treatment at Hazelden there are a certain number of Roman Catholic patients who have what I call a "Killer Nun Story" ("I went to parochial school. There was a nun. She was nine feet tall and had a tire iron . . ."). Because they have a "Killer Nun Story" they close the door on the Catholic Church, God, Jesus, a Higher Power, the "Big Book" of A.A., sponsorship, the whole deal: out. In contrast, there are other patients with a Roman Catholic heritage that is inert, because they have been drinking and using drugs. They decide to ride the van and go to a friendly Roman Catholic church for the Sacrament of Reconciliation and for the mass. They discover themes like forgiveness and grace, beauty, community, serenity, reconciliation, the presence of God, and they think, "Hey! There's something here I can use." It's the same religion, but it could help or hinder their spirituality, according to the quality and nature of the relationships and the type of experience they are having.

■ SPIRITUALITY VERSUS RELIGION

Another difference between spirituality and religion is that all religions come with a claim of truth, that basically goes like this: "The truth exists, whether you believe it or not. We, who know what the truth is, are prepared to reveal it to you, if you will participate in our religion." They then disagree about what the truth is. In western religions, the truth consists of a set of facts. "Jesus Christ is the Son of God, Savior." "There is one God, and Mohammed is His Prophet." "Israel is God's chosen people." Those are all factual statements. In eastern religions, the truth is less a set of facts and more a process of enlightenment, or growing into the truth. Both types of religions are concerned with truth. Religions have a body of doctrine and many have creeds that are to be recited, accepted, and aspired to.

■ EXPERIENCE, STRENGTH, AND HOPE

Religion is rooted in a vision of ultimate truth. Spirituality is rooted in experience. The Twelve Step programs, and other support groups such as cancer support or grief support, are spiritual, rather than religious. They do not hold a truth one must accept or a body of doctrine to be received and accepted. Instead, they propose to share their experience, strength, and hope to solve common living problems. They are rooted in the experience of their members, rather than the doctrine of either religion or another discipline.

In Twelve Step meetings, people share their experience, strength, and hope. Some of this is spiritual experience. They share their problems and concerns and report on how they prayed, meditated, read their program literature, and talked to their sponsors. Participants have a choice. As they listen, if it is rubbish, they leave it there. If, however, it sounds promising, they pick it up, take it home, and try it out. If it works, they keep doing it. They build their spirituality starting with what other people have reported from their spiritual experience, what they have tried, and what they have found effective for solving life problems. There is no need to take anything on faith. All that is required is an openness to living life according to spiritual principles, and the willingness to research how well it works. They start with what sounds plausible, and keep those elements of spirituality that actually work for them.

■ THE ULTIMATE TEST

An example of testing something that comes from a group experience is from my own chronic illness of alcoholism. At the end of chapter three in the "Big Book," *Alcoholics Anonymous*, the author states, "The alcoholic at certain times has no effective mental defense against the first drink. Except in a few rare cases, neither he nor any other human being can provide such a defense. His defense must come from a Higher Power."[2] I had read this many times, and certainly did not disagree with it. However, it wasn't until the summer of 1997 that it came true for me.

I had a phone call at 10:30 p.m. from my older sister, inviting me to drop everything and fly down south at full fare for a weekend of family craziness. I declined, on the idea that I don't have to attend every argument to which I am invited. But when I got off the phone, I really wanted to drink right then. The local Twelve Step meetings were over by that hour. My wife wasn't home. I called a couple of people on my phone list, but I didn't feel any better. So I said to God, "Remember that part at the end of chapter three, where it says 'no effective mental defense' and 'must rely on a Higher Power'? Well, you're on!" Miraculously, I immediately felt better. I now believe in that passage much more firmly. Before, it was good insight from A.A. in the 1930s. Now it is my own.

This is an example of the Third Step in Twelve Step programs: "We made a decision to turn our will and our lives over to the care of God *as we understood Him.*" In that moment, I was turning over my will (my thoughts on drinking) and my life (my actions) over to God's care. I know of people with other chronic illnesses who are doing the same thing. Cancer patients sometimes visualize themselves being touched, healed, or cared for by God. Patients headed for surgery often consciously turn over the outcome to God.

■ WORKING TOGETHER

Religion and spirituality are not in competition, but they are different. Anyone can have both a spiritual program and a religion. Ideally, they will enhance each other. There is a cliche that states: "Religion is for those who are afraid of going to hell, and spirituality is for those who have already been there." This slogan sets up spirituality as better than religion. People who haven't "been to hell" and are not afraid of going there may well be very happy in both a religion and a spiritually healthy way of life.

■ THE FIFTH STEP: MOVING TOWARDS RECOVERY

Because A.A. uses the language of Christianity in its "Big Book," there is a natural confusion that it is Christianity. People assume they are the same because of this resemblance. This is particularly evident around the Fifth Step: "We admitted to God, to ourselves, and to another human being the exact nature of our wrongs." This is easily confused with Christian confession. They are, however, entirely distinct. They have a different purpose and outcome.

Christianity has to do with sin and salvation and the goal is salvation. The focus of Twelve Step programs like A.A. and Narcotics Anonymous (N.A.) is addiction and recovery and the goal is recovery. In Christianity, one can be saved or lost. In recovery, one can be "drunk" (high, codependent, etc.) or "sober" (clean, sane, etc.). Considering both salvation and recovery for the alcoholic, there are four possible outcomes: sober and saved; sober and lost, saved but drunk, and both drunk and lost. A Christian alcoholic who wishes to be both sober and saved can work both the Christian faith and the program of A.A. for success.

In Christian confession, the problem of sin is solved by confession and the forgiveness of God that follows. In the Fifth Step, the problem of wrongdoing is identified, but not solved. There are more steps. Freedom from the effects of the wrongs comes as the result of Steps Six through Nine. Confession moves one towards salvation. The Fifth Step moves one towards recovery. Both can be of value, but they are not the same in either purpose or outcome.

■ DEFINITION OF A HIGHER POWER

It is not necessary to believe in a Higher Power to benefit from a spiritually healthy way of life. It is necessary to develop a Higher Power relationship so that there is something outside of us that is improving our spirit. I have a suggested minimum standard for a Higher Power. It has three elements: (1) It's not me. (2) It's more powerful than me. (3) It wants to help me. It is said that you can have anything as your Higher Power, even a Styrofoam cup or a light bulb. However, these do not meet my suggested standard. I have never actually met someone who was getting help for life from a Styrofoam cup or light bulb. I suggest looking as high as possible for a Higher Power.

■ THE HIGHER POWER ENCOUNTER

There are three levels on which this Higher Power can be encountered: (1) A Twelve Step or other support group. (2) A recovery program as a whole. (3) An intangible Higher Power. I can get help from my home group in my Twelve Step program. In it, I find a room full of consultants who are walking the same path as I. There is also a migraine headache support group where I live. They know the problem, their program and they know me. I can take any problem or concern to the group and get help. The group can be my Higher Power. In time, we discover that behind the group there is another form of this power called the program. I can travel to a different place or a different culture, but if it is my program I will find the same Higher Power there. I've been to meetings on an island off the coast of Maine that has 37 year-round residents, two meetings a week, and they need them. There, the human race is divided into "islanders" and "people from away." Even though I am a person "from away" I fit right in the first time I went, because it was my program. In time, most people, but not everyone, come to believe in an intangible Higher Power that they call God, Higher Power, or another name. It is possible to connect with a Higher Power at any time in any or all of these forms. People who don't believe in God can have a lifetime of recovery by connecting at the group or program level.

■ SELF-DEFINITION

Before clinicians attempt to understand their patient's spirituality, they may wish to start with their own spirituality. They should begin with their own story which includes their family of origin. Many of their core beliefs about life, about themselves, about trust, and about a Higher Power are formed very early. Much of this formation happens before they even have words to shape their thoughts. After all, they are not born "hard wired" for the human race. They are born knowing how to eat, sleep, defecate, smile when amused, scream when annoyed, and that's about it. They learn who they are, and begin the process of self-definition, by seeing themselves reflected in the faces of people around them.

■ MIRACLE BABIES

I have two grandchildren who I refer to as "the miracle babies" because they were born to parents who are married, love each other, are not chemically dependent, and want children. They arrived in the world and saw big faces that smiled at each of them and said, "You're the most beautiful baby in the entire world. You're intelligent, loved, and life is grand." So they brightened up and came to expect that life was trustworthy and good. Other children who receive other messages from the large faces in their world reach other conclusions.

■ TRUSTING IN OTHERS

People set their trust levels by how trustworthy the world is when they're children. Perceptions can always be changed later based on new information, but original perceptions are set very near origins. Two-year-olds can be observed standing still and screaming at the top of their lungs for no readily apparent reason. They are "testing the smoke detector" to see if anybody comes in response to their cry of alarm. If no one listens and no one cares, they become insecure. Once they know the signal works, they grow out of the habit of testing it.

There is also a tendency for people's beliefs about a Higher Power to resemble their childhood beliefs about their parents. This is because when they're little, their parents are big. If they went home one evening and there was a fourteen-foot tall, nine hundred pound person saying "Straighten up and fly right!" they'd probably try, because the giant is big. If they had warm, loving, nurturing parents, they may end up with a Higher Power who's like a cosmic muffin. If they had harsh, perfectionist, critical parents, they may end up with Thor, the thunder god, waiting to strike them with a lightning bolt if they do one little thing wrong. It's worthwhile to begin to separate their image of a Higher Power from their parental or cultural expectations, because their parents and culture are only people, not God.

The most common cultural image of God in society is that of the judge: an old man with a ledger book. On the left side is everything they've done wrong and on the right side is everything they've done right. Someday He will draw the line, add it all up, and judge them. Two problems exist with this image: (1) It may not be true. (2) It's scary, resulting in people trying to hide from their Higher Power.

■ BEING SATISFIED WITH LIFE

A reexamination of one's Higher Power understanding is useful for recovery. Recovery for the chronically ill means successful management of their illness in a way that patients are satisfied with their life. Instead of the judge, the Twelve Step programs offer an understanding of a Higher Power that is characterized by restoration and care. Step Two speaks of coming to believe in a power greater than themselves that could restore them to sanity. Step Three speaks of making a decision to turn their will and their lives over to the care of God, as they understand God. Restoration and care are integral parts of how the program understands God.

■ SPIRITUAL ISSUES

As people consider their childhood and original families, they can discover their spiritual issues. Spiritual issues are simply themes or metaphors that keep reemerging in their lives, that either enhance their relationships with Higher Power, self, and others, or block those relationships. These themes often operate outside their awareness, and produce consistent results. Both positive and negative spiritual issues emerge from their stories.

Some positive spiritual issues include love, comfort, trust, honesty, openness, willingness, a sense of community, compassion, hope, a desire to be of service, and a dedication to reality. These all enhance relationships.

Some negative spiritual issues include fear, distrust, abandonment, hostility and contempt towards others, dishonesty, a closed and unwilling spirit, isolation, grandiosity, denial, and despair or hopelessness. These all separate people from their Higher Power, other people, and keep them from being comfortable with themselves.

Once spiritual issues are identified, they try to enhance the positives by deliberately practicing them on a daily basis. They confront the negative ones with changed behavior on that topic, until the negative spiritual issues lose their power. They start by changing their behavior because feelings are hard to change. Attitudes may or may not change, depending on their skill at noticing how their attitudes are affecting their feelings. However, their behavior is always within reach. As they change their behavior, the tyranny of their negative spiritual issues goes away. The issues themselves may not be entirely absent from their lives, but they no longer have the power to dominate their days.

■ MAKING CHANGES: BETWEEN HOPE AND DESPAIR

A frequent spiritual issue in chronic illness is the continuum between despair and hope. Robert was a physician who pushed very hard. He worked long, hard hours in a research laboratory, played squash aggressively, and carried on a couple of romances at a time, disguising each relationship from the other woman. He took out his aggressions on his staff. They in turn began to sabotage his work.

Although Robert had chest pains and sweats, he acted as if he didn't have a heart problem. He tried to will it away, just as he exerted his will in other areas of life, usually successfully. This time was different though. When he couldn't get his chest to stop hurting, he sought medical treatment and was scheduled for bypass surgery. Post surgery, he went into an emotional slump. He despaired about his life ever being good again. He stopped dating, his research work was desultory, and he avoided even modest exercise. His clergyman made a comment to him that made an impact. He said, "To feel normal, act normal." It was suggested that his despair might be fed by his inaction. He was to behave as if he had hope for a good life, even after a bypass. A list of things he could do was made including: definite hours for work, moderate exercise, treating his staff with dignity and respect, and resuming a friendship with one of the women he really liked.

Robert's changed behavior helped restore his hope. He traded long hours in the lab for a 30-hour a week clinical practice, treated the staff there well, and dated one woman without subterfuge.

Behaving in a hopeful way made him hopeful and gave him better cardiac health, as well.

■ SPIRITUALITY AND CHILD ABUSE

It is possible to change negative spiritual issues by changing behavior even in cases of extreme damage. Alan was struggling as an adult with the effects of childhood abuse. He came from a history of alcoholism and violence. From his life experiences of paying the price in his body for other people's violence and rage came his major spiritual issues: fear and abandonment. As a child, his fear was for the next time he would be beaten. If his mother beat him badly enough, his father would dump him off at the hospital like a pile of bloody laundry, and he'd be picked up again when he was discharged, but no one would come to visit him. That created the sense of abandonment.

From a psychological viewpoint, he was diagnosed with Post-Traumatic Stress Disorder. From a spiritual viewpoint, he had come to believe that God would not help him. He lived life from a viewpoint of vigilance and self-reliance. His defenses protected him well from danger. The spiritual issues of fear and abandonment led him to be afraid of most things, and to never rely on other people.

To confront his fear and sense of abandonment, he began to break through the isolation that was the logical consequence of it. He sought connections, through psychotherapy, Al-Anon for adult children of alcoholics, spiritual direction, and by talking with his wife and a few friends about the reality of trauma. He also began to break through his fear. His fears had grown and generalized. He loved to travel, but was afraid to fly. He took flying lessons and got a student pilot's license, which allowed him to fly a plane alone. He took the initiative to apply for a job that he wanted a great deal, and then stepped forward offering to take on new tasks and responsibilities, even though he had a fear of failure and rejection. Gradually he became less isolated and afraid. As of now, he is still taking on new ventures, partly on their own merit, and partly to overcome his negative spiritual issues.

■ A "GOD CONCEPT"

It is also possible to re-imagine one's Higher Power, in a way that fits one's particular spiritual needs. I'm not suggesting that we make one up. We need a real Higher Power, not a fictional one. However, every image or understanding of a Higher Power is inadequate and incomplete, because of the relatively small size of our brains. If we're going to be inaccurate, and can only know God "through a glass, darkly" then we might as well have a "God concept" that matches our spiritual needs.

■ FLEXIBLE GOD RELATIONSHIPS

Some women have been sexually abused by their fathers and have difficulty saying a prayer that begins "Our Father, who art in heaven ..." It's the wrong image, and casts God in the form of their abuser. They may be happier with a female image of God and with the Serenity Prayer.

One of Alan's images of a Higher Power is a color that printers call "non-photo blue." It doesn't turn up well on photocopiers. This is because one of his symptoms of a scrambled brain is seeing a light orange color where it doesn't really exist, from time to time. The opposite of that orange is non-photo blue, which represents for him healing, kindness, and care, all of which he needs from his Higher Power. Another image of his Higher Power is represented by a sense of touch, or of being held. There's no picture related to that image at all, just kindly touch. When he was hospitalized for a while, unable to see, touch became very important.

Over the centuries, the Roman Catholic Church has intuited the need for flexibility in relationships with God. If people feel awkward talking to God, they may choose to talk to the Virgin Mary, or the patron saint of their nationality or occupational group. Mexicans often feel much better talking to the brown-skinned Lady of Guadalupe than talking to a blue-eyed Jesus.

Several images or understandings of a Higher Power are possible. For people who have no image or understanding at all, praying "to whom it may concern", or just praying to the air might be appropriate. The very act of prayer puts us in a frame of mind and spirit to be open to a Higher Power relationship.

■ A SPIRITUAL AWAKENING

I recall a Hazelden patient, John, who had no Higher Power, and who was very annoying to his peers in treatment. He constantly found fault with them and the treatment facility. He had heard my suggestion about talking to the air. He was facing a "peer evaluation" in which his peers would assess his recovery and treatment progress. The evaluation was likely to be harsh. He went outside and said to the air, "If I'm going to have a spiritual awakening, I better have one now, because they're going to kill me!" Remarkably, he did have a spiritual awakening. Suddenly, his negativity was replaced with gratitude for life, and kindness toward his peers. He became aware that he was an addict and that treatment was a wonderful opportunity. In the peer evaluation the next day, every one of the 19 men there noted his changed attitude. He still didn't have a name for his Higher Power, but he was aware of being changed for the better by a power greater than himself. I ran into John shortly after his peer evaluation. Although I knew nothing of his prayer to the air, I immediately noticed both happiness and a lightness of spirit about him.

■ SPIRITUAL AWAKENINGS: THE TWELFTH STEP

There are two kinds of spiritual awakenings: sudden and gradual. First, only a few people get sudden spiritual awakenings. It is a kind of calling card from their Higher Power saying "I'm real." There are two problems with this: most people don't get them, and they sometimes go away as quickly as they came. The second kind is the slowly developing spiritual awakening, which both William James in his book *The Varieties of Religious Experience*[3] and A.A. call "the educational variety." This is available to anyone who will work a program of spiritual growth. The last step of A.A. Twelve Steps reads: "Having had a spiritual awakening as the result of these steps, we

> ### ■ CHEMICAL DEPENDENCY: A MODEL FOR THE SUCCESSFUL MANAGEMENT OF OTHER CHRONIC ILLNESSES
>
> I am a Christian, and a United Methodist Minister. I also find other revelations about the nature of God in other religions. Christianity, with some additional insights from other religions, is my model for religion. Because I am an alcoholic and drug addict, I have had the opportunity to use the Twelve Steps in several different programs, and have found them to be an effective treatment both for addiction and for spiritual bankruptcy. The Twelve Steps have become my model for spiritual growth, and I cheerfully recommend them to people who have any religion or no religion, any recovery issue or none. Understanding addiction, or chemical dependency, gives insight into many other chronic illnesses.
>
> I call chemical dependency a disease because it can be reliably diagnosed with a standard set of criteria, follows a predictable course, responds to treatment, and can be both progressive and fatal if not successfully treated. It can serve as a model for the successful management of other chronic illnesses.

tried to carry this message to other alcoholics, and to practice these principles in all our affairs." The spiritual awakening is the result of the steps, not a qualification for embarking on them.

Chemical Dependency

■ SPIRITUALITY AND RELATIONSHIPS

Chemical dependency is a spiritual disease, an emotional disease, a mental disease, and a physical disease. The progression of the disease is first spiritual, then emotional, mental, and finally physical. The progression of recovery is the reverse.

Spirituality consists of the quality and nature of people's relationships in three dimensions: with a Higher Power, with themselves, and with other people. One common effect, early in the

progression of a chronic illness, is that their spirituality deterio-
rates, whether or not they have a belief in God.

Sober teenagers in love are very spiritual people. They are
intensely interested in relationships and will sit with the telephone
glued to their ears for hours, just listening to their loved ones
breathe. When any of them are courting in a sober way, they take
an intense interest in the other person, in themselves, and in life
itself. When they are trying to get someone to marry them or
make a commitment to them, they will sit up late at night for
hours. They will talk about everything including: life, death, meaning, purpose, vocation, marriage, family, children, where they
want to live, education, retirement, religion, God, and all of their
plans together.

■ A MULTIPLE CHOICE TEST

The pull of chronic illness is that it begins to absorb attentions.
Gradually thoughts and feelings can center around the illness instead
of centering on life, love, and relationships. The intangibles fade out
of life: love, honor, trust, comfort, hope, compassion, and curiosity.
Life is reduced to a multiple choice test:

"Are you home?" (a) yes (b) no.

"Are you hungry?" (a) yes (b) no.

"Whadda you want?" (a) pizza (b) Chinese (c) leftovers (d) I've got
some frozen chicken breasts I could thaw out and fry up.

"Do you want to do something this evening?" (a) television (b) rent a
video (c) I don't care (d) let's go to bed early.

As we get sicker, life is reduced another notch to grunt, shrug, or
meaningless gesture:

"Are you home?" "Uh."

"Are you hungry?" "Uhhhh."

"Whadda you want?" "I dunno."

"Do you want to do something this evening?" "Eyah."

They're not physically gone or divorced, but nothing is happening in their relationship. They are spiritually sick at home.

■ THE CHRONICALLY ILL AND RELATIONSHIPS

People also get spiritually sick at work. The chronically ill who previously went to work and had fun and were creative now treat work as drudgery and might make the following statements:

> "Oh, God, it's Monday." "Thank God it's Friday." "The only difference between this place and the Titanic is that the Titanic had a band." "I can only please one person a day, and today's not your day. Tomorrow's not looking good either."

When they allow a chronic illness to set the tone for their days, they become spiritually sick.

■ SPIRITUALLY SICK AT THE BALLPARK

We can be spiritually sick even when we're doing things we allegedly enjoy. I like to go to the wildly popular Saint Paul Saints baseball games, a very minor league team that's a lot of fun. In the stands, they have face painting, massages, and haircuts. Silly contests take place between the innings. I get to see some of "Hazelden's future customers" there, fans with a beer in each hand. There's even a vendor with a cell phone. You can call in your seat location lest you be forced to watch a moment without a beer. The fascinating thing about the heavy drinkers is that they are angry for much of the game. A batter misses, and they shout "whatssamatterwityou!." They are spiritually sick at the ball park.

■ THE DOMINEERING CHRONIC ILLNESS

The father of one of my good friends began to focus more and more on his illnesses. He was older, had aches and pains, and claimed some chest pains and shortness of breath. He would go to a family outing or event, but rather than focusing on the experience, he would zero-in on how sick he felt. This would make him restless and irritable, and he would want to leave before others. If they didn't want to leave yet, he'd develop chest pains, forcing an exit. His relationships and his activities were dominated by his illnesses. When he died, I suggested a tombstone epitaph of "I TOLD you I was sick!"

■ TAKING IT OUT ON SOMEONE ELSE

Under the influence of chronic illness, people can become emotionally sick. They may have unhealthy emotions. Depression appears to have a physiological basis, but it is experienced as a flat feeling and a sense of purposelessness. The emotional range available to the depressed patient is limited. Chronic pain also can make the patient snappish. Years ago, there was a successful series of television ads for an analgesic. The older woman in the ads would snap at her adult daughter. The daughter would say "Mother! Sure, you have a headache. But don't take it out on me!" This was a sufficiently universal experience that the expression made it into the common language of the time. A diabetic with too little sugar gets irritable and one with too much sugar gets sleepy. A cancer patient who experiences alternating signs of relapse and remission may alternate between hope and despair, anger and happiness. People addicted to alcohol or drugs experience predictable disorders of mood or affect.

■ HOW SICK ARE YOU?

As chronic illness progresses, people can become mentally ill; in the sense of having thought disorders. They think things that are not true, and facts do not break through their denial. When I was visiting in the hospital as a parish pastor, I would routinely ask the patient "How sick are you?" Frequently I would already have that information, and be aware that they had it too, but I wanted to hear their response to the question. Sometimes patients with life threatening illnesses, who were well informed, would insist that they were just fine.

> Sometimes people who were being sent home from the hospital because there was no effective treatment available would distort this information believing that they were going home because they were well now.

■ DISTORTING THE SYMPTOMS OF DISEASE

Alcoholics and addicts tend to distort the symptoms of their disease and reinterpret them as someone else's defects or errors. An alcoholic who keeps getting arrested for drunken driving may distort their legal problems into a politically motivated trend towards prohibition. It becomes the police officer's fault, rather than a sign that addiction is getting out of control.

Physical damage tends to come late in the process, which feeds their denial: "If my eyeballs aren't yellow yet, I'm not sick at all!"

There are four dimensions of disease which include: spiritual, emotional, mental, and physical. The most common form of recovery is physical recovery first, mental second, emotional third, and finally spiritual. For a patient with a serious illness, when they physically recover, their thinking tends to become less agitated and more settled, their feelings become more benign, and their spirits are lifted. The problem with this natural progression towards healing and wholeness is that, for chronic illness patients, they may not be physically healed. This is the heart of the problem: Is mental, emotional, and spiritual health dependent on physical healing? Probably not. By applying spiritual principles to patient's lives, they can become well in mind, emotions, and spirit, even while still being physically ill. Practicing these principles may also ameliorate their physical illnesses, as well.

■ PRACTICING THE TWELVE STEPS

To understand how these principles work, a brief overview of how to work the Twelve Steps[4] in order to recover as an alcoholic and drug addict is provided. As these principles are reviewed in the coming chapters, they will be linked to the treatment of other chronic illnesses, and to the development of satisfactory lives, regardless of the patient's physical conditions.

■ STEP ONE: HONESTY

Step One reads "We admitted we were powerless over alcohol and our lives had become unmanageable." (N.A. says, "powerless over addiction," Survivors of Incest Anonymous says, "powerless over the incest experience," and other programs substitute another phrase here.)

Step One calls for the spiritual principle of honesty. To recover as an alcoholic and addict, people must admit that they actually are addicted. However, mere admission does not move them forward towards recovery. Step One provides good information, but does not produce change by itself.

■ STEP TWO: HOPE

Hope is introduced in Step Two. It reads: "We came to believe that a power greater than ourselves could restore us to sanity." This hope is developed by attending Twelve Step meetings. People come to believe that a power greater than themselves can restore them to sanity by watching other people getting well. This is why they need meetings: They need to see other people's lives changing in order to give them hope and encouragement to embark on this process of change for themselves.

■ STEP THREE: FAITH

Step Three involves faith. It reads: "We made a decision to turn our will and our lives over to the care of God as we understood Him." From observing other people's recovery, they make a decision that they want what others have and are willing to go to any lengths to get it. Because others have made this decision and it is working well for them, others follow too. Some people are reluctant to take Step Three because they are afraid to turn their will and their lives over to the care of God. However, the Step calls only for a decision.

Anyone can make a decision. The decision comes true in the process of doing Steps Four through Eleven. The full benefits of Step Twelve are then received.

■ STEP FOUR: COURAGE

Having made that decision, they can tell God that they want to turn their will and life over to Him. This takes courage. God says, "Now here's your homework, Step Four: 'We made a searching and fearless moral inventory of ourselves.' You've taken everyone else's inventory, now take your own."

■ WHAT COURAGE INVOLVES

The spiritual principle of Step Four is courage. I avoided the step for a time by noting that I still had fear, and was thus not fearless. I finally realized that courage does not consist of the absence of fear, but rather of doing the right thing even when afraid.

■ STEP FIVE: INTEGRITY

Integrity is practiced by taking the Fifth Step: "We admitted to God, to ourselves, and to another human being the exact nature of our wrongs." Integrity has to do with wholeness. Reporting only successes and admirable points will not make a person whole. When people include discreditable parts of their lives in their stories, then they become more whole.

Taking the Fifth Step does not correct wrongs, it identifies them. Some people are disappointed with their Fifth Step, because they do not feel wonderful. This euphoric feeling comes after the successful completion of Step Nine. A Fifth Step is diagnosis, not treatment.

■ STEP SIX: WILLINGNESS

Step Six brings willingness to have God change them: "We became entirely ready to have God remove these defects of character." This is not a self-help program. Self-help for chemical dependency is a myth: it's about as effective as tickling oneself. It seems, conceptually, like it ought to work, but nothing happens. People can only be tickled in relationships. They only recover in a network of relationships with peers, programs, and Higher Powers. In this step, they become ready to have God change them, rather than setting out on a program to correct their own defects. One way that God changes them is by leading them through the rest of the Steps.

■ STEP SEVEN: HUMILITY

Step Seven calls for humility. "We humbly asked Him to remove our shortcomings." When people are ready to have God remove their defects of character, they join in this step with millions of men and women who are taking this path. Humility has nothing to do with humiliation. It means having an appropriate view of themselves, neither grandiose nor ashamed. Humility means living in right relationships with their Higher Power, themselves, and others. In regard to God, humility means being clear about which one of them actually is God. When they try to run their lives, and handle their own chemical dependency through self-will, they are playing God. They are underqualified for the role, and it doesn't work out.

The authors of the Twelve Steps go to some lengths to avoid repeating a phrase. The "wrongs" in Step Five become "defects of character" in Step Six and "shortcomings" in Step Seven. In addition to the literary device of avoiding the same phrase, this also represents the spiritual progress experienced in the Steps. As progress is made, wrongs soften into character defects and finally shortcomings. What's wrong with people is gradually losing its power to determine the course of their lives.

■ STEP EIGHT: COMPASSION

Step Eight is characterized by the spiritual principle of compassion. People prepare to reconcile wherever possible with others by taking this Step: "We made a list of all persons we had harmed, and became willing to make amends to them all." Instead of dividing the world into people they like and people they dislike, they begin to practice the principle of anonymity and become willing to make amends to people whether they like them or not.

To get a good list, three sets of people need to be included: those harmed on purpose, those harmed by accident, and those harmed by omission. Whether or not they had a "good reason" doesn't enter into this list making process. All that is necessary is to inventory the people whom they have harmed.

Once their list is complete, there is another part to this Step: becoming willing to make amends to them all. This involves a change of character. Maybe they're not willing. Maybe they're looking for a chance to harm others again. A small scale example of this is office gossip and politics: Are they willing to let go of gossip, criticism, and revenge as a way of life at work? This Step involves a change whereby they become harmless people.

■ STEP NINE: JUSTICE

Step Nine brings justice back into life: "We made direct amends wherever possible, except when to do so would injure them or others." Step Nine should be taken when they're well established in their recovery, and in the habit of being guided both by their Higher Power and by trusted sponsors. They take their amends list and carefully plan out what the appropriate amends would be. If making direct amends would bring harm to them or others, they move to indirect amends. They should include themselves in the list of "others." That is, if making direct amends would harm them (not merely embarrass or cost them money) then they do not make them.

Indirect amends are always possible, and may be ultimately more important than direct amends. Indirect amends consist of first changing behavior on that issue, and ultimately involves changing their character with the help of peers, programs, and a Higher Power. Amends have relatively little to do with apologies. When people amend a law, they change its meaning. They don't merely apologize for passing it. For example, if they have stolen money, the direct amends is to pay it back. The indirect amends is to stop stealing money, and to move beyond that to complete financial honesty and integrity.

The "Big Book," *Alcoholics Anonymous*, states that if they are painstaking with this phase of their development, they are going to know a new freedom and a new happiness, and the promises of recovery will come true.

■ MY FAVORITE PROMISE

My favorite promise is that "we will intuitively know how to handle situations which used to baffle us." After completing Step Nine, we feel really well because we are getting well.

■ STEP TEN: PERSEVERANCE

To hold onto the gains made in the first nine Steps, perseverance is practiced with Step Ten: "We continued to take personal inventory, and when we were wrong, promptly admitted it." Initially, this can be a daily inventory. As people grow in the program, it can become a continual theme. Most of their wrongs can be caught within moments of committing them. This self-examination works in much the same way as the spelling checker on word processing software does, placing a red line under words that are misspelled.

■ IT GOES IN PHASES

My experience has shown that it goes in phases. First, I notice that I have done something wrong after I have done it and after the consequences have appeared. Then I begin to notice that I am doing something wrong while in the process of doing it. After practice, I notice that I am about to do something wrong, but I do it anyway. Further along in my development, I notice that I am about to do something wrong, and avoid doing it. Finally, I don't even want to do it. This process is not complete, but I persevere in it.

■ STEP ELEVEN: SPIRITUAL AWARENESS

Step Eleven focuses on spiritual awareness. "We sought through prayer and meditation to improve our conscious contact with God as we understand Him, praying only for knowledge of God's will for our lives and the power to carry that out." People don't typically wait to begin prayer and meditation until Step Eleven, but spiritual awareness comes more fully and naturally after the first Ten Steps have been taken. Most people have prayed before recovery while others have meditated. This Step suggests what to pray for: both knowledge and power. Experience reveals that there have been many times when they knew what to do, but lacked the power to carry it out.

■ STEP TWELVE: SERVICE

Step Twelve sums up the results of doing the first Eleven Steps: "Having had a spiritual awakening as the result of these steps, we tried to carry this message to alcoholics (addicts in N.A.) and to practice these principles in all our affairs." The spiritual principle is service. There is no evidence that an eleven and a half step program works: "Having had a spiritual awakening as the result of these steps, I'm out of here!" Recovery is a spiritual gift from a Higher Power. If they do not care to pass on the gift, they may not get to keep it. That's how this works. It is in carrying the message to the next person that their own recovery is assured.

■ A SPIRITUAL AWAKENING

Spiritual well being is the most likely aspect of recovery to be overlooked, because it comes last. Many people find that they feel well enough part way along the Twelve Step path, and do not fully live the Steps. They may be physically alcohol and drug free, mentally accurate, and even emotionally stable enough to satisfy themselves and those around them. By stopping short of a spiritual awakening, they miss much of the fun of recovery.

Approaches to chronic illness often have the same limitations. Some approaches focus only on physical health while others will include mental and emotional health. Healthy spirituality is a vital part of healing for chronic illness. It not only completes healing, but may also influence physical, mental, and emotional health in positive ways.

In the balance of this book, the universal spiritual principles that formed the basis of the Twelve Steps will be examined. How those principles can give spiritual fitness, resilience, and good lives will be seen. How patients with chronic illnesses can apply these principles to their lives, and how the principles can inform clinical practices will be thoroughly examined. In the next chapter, Bowen White, a medical doctor, provides a unique perspective of spirituality in the treatment of patients with chronic illness.

REFERENCES

1. "Alternative Medicine Man," *Discover Magazine*, August 1999, pp. 56–58.
2. *Alcoholics Anonymous*, 3rd ed., Alcoholics Anonymous World Services, Inc., New York, 1976, p. 43.
3. W. James, *The Varieties of Religious Experience*, Random House, New York, 1999.
4. *Alcoholics Anonymous*, pp. 59–60.

3

Chapter Three

Spirituality and Chronic Illness

Bowen F. White

Spirituality is an integral, influential part of most people's lives that defines much of who they are. Yet this non-scientific dimension is often ignored in patient care. In modern medical care, physical and spiritual components reside in two different worlds. By taking the time to understand how patients with chronic illness view themselves and their world, clinicians can guide them to discover meaning in their suffering and thereby improve their well-being. Deeper contact with patients allows clinicians to be with their patients in a way that offers comfort and the opportunity for healing even though a cure may not be available.

There is no scientific evidence that humans possess a spiritual component. After all, it is not quantifiable and does not fit on a slide for histologic examination. Yet studies have shown that about 95 percent of humans have a spiritual belief system. A belief in a spiritual reality does not necessarily mean that a person follows a specific religious persuasion or attends religious services regularly. It does mean that most patients have an interest, at some level, in non-scientific areas that help explain how they view themselves and the world. It is vitally important to understand how patients see things if clinicians are to serve them effectively. By ignoring the patient's beliefs, clinicians are not treating the whole person.

What Is Chronic Illness?

Chronic illnesses, defined here as maladies that cannot be cured, will not be limited to a narrow spectrum of problems. When people are suffering from a chronic illness, they often confront their mortality. They no longer have the luxury of ignoring their physical, mental, and emotional state. Over time, denial yields to the unavoidable reality of disease and the realization that both health and life are transient. Sooner or later, both are lost—a scary proposition for most mortals, regardless of spiritual beliefs.

The treatment of chronically ill patients produces chronic discomfort for many physicians. Medical training focuses more on providing cures for acute problems through surgical and medicinal interventions, or the conventional "fix it" model of care. But even though interventions for an acute problem may also alleviate an acute exacerbation of a chronic problem, the underlying infirmity usually is incurable. For example, someone with chronic heart disease may receive angioplasty or heart bypass surgery for an acute exacerbation such as a myocardial infarction. Or a patient with diabetes may require acute surgical and medical treatment for a foot infection that is accompanied by gangrene and osteomyelitis. Is the patient cured of heart disease following angioplasty? If so, why is the procedure repeated frequently for many patients? Is the diabetic patient cured of diabetes by intensive wound management?

In today's culture of youth orientation and obsession with the superficiality of youth maintenance, the flashlight of our individual and collective attention shines on the superficial. That is, until chronic illness stops people short and brings into focus those things they had ignored below the surface. Then people may see the familiar with new eyes, and, instead of taking themselves and other people for granted, they feel a new sense of gratitude for their lives and the people in them. The patient and perhaps even the family may then recognize the value of the illness.

■ IF IT AIN'T BROKE, DON'T FIX IT

In my medical practice, I try to create a respectful environment for my patients that allows them to find meaning in their illness by looking deeper into their lives. Don't get me wrong. I don't think that we have to wait for some significant life event to wake us from our ordinary state of awareness. But, let's face it. "If it ain't broke, don't fix it" is the cultural norm. Some people do not need a significant event alarm to leave the bed of cultural and spiritual slumber, but they are an anomaly.

Let's examine our lives. What do you see? I know I can be slow on the uptake, and sometimes need an attention-getting crisis to break the status quo. For example, as a ninth grader, my grades were poor and I was frequently in trouble. Basketball was my only salvation, but a knee injury in mid-December kept me from finishing the season. This stirred feelings of inadequacy because my self-worth was grounded in the external world, in my accomplishments on the basketball court, not in a more solid, inner sense of well-being. Most of my grades dropped to D's and F's. While I tore up my report cards to keep the bad news from my parents, eventually they found out and hired a tutor named Mr. Berg. He knew what basketball meant to me, and after our algebra sessions, we would shoot baskets. I was accustomed to adults who treated me as if I were a problem, but in this new, trusting atmosphere, I felt comfortable expressing my feelings of confusion and fear. Mr. Berg didn't focus on the scared kid that I was, but treated me like the person I could become, honoring something latent that had not yet found expression. With Mr. Berg's help, I began to see myself differently.

Crises in our lives interrupt the ordinary routine of daily survival so that living fully becomes an option. We replace a take-it-for-granted spirit with an attitude of gratitude, denial with acceptance, and a psychology of scarcity with a psychology of abundance. In short, we see the familiar in new ways. And when I look back on the event that precipitated this shift in awareness, I am grateful it occurred.

Paul Azinger, a professional golfer and former PGA champion, did a television interview one year after his diagnosis of lymphoma. When asked how he felt about the experience he said, "Having cancer was the best thing that ever happened to me." His cancer altered his life, preventing him from continuing activities that had made him successful. Success itself now had new meaning. Like Paul, there are patients who are grateful for their world-stopping illnesses.

Because of the enviable opportunities in the US, people are acculturated to go for the American Dream, to "grab the brass ring," or "to be all you can be." It is frequently said that the secret to success is hard work. People are told they can do whatever they desire if they are willing to pay the price in hard work. So, they learn to shine the flashlight of their attention on their work. It defines them. People give energy to those things that get their attention. Shine a flashlight into a dark closet and all that will be seen is what is illuminated. A significant world-stopping illness often compels people to begin looking around the darkened spaces of their own interior closets. While focusing on their inner selves, they see what may have been there all along, while they were busily attending to other things. The light of their attention bathes the neglected parts of them. Once their priorities shift, energy can flow toward what they deem significant—not what was most important to their parents or culture.

A contemporary tale of shifting priorities is vividly described in the best-selling book, *Tuesdays with Morrie* by Mitch Albom.[1] Mitch, a sports writer for the Detroit Free Press, was living a very busy, successful programmed existence here in the Excited States of America. Then, he had a world-stopping event—not through a chronic illness but by accidentally seeing Ted Koppel interview a man dying of ALS, Lou Gehrig's disease, on Nightline. The patient was none other than Morrie Schwartz, Mitch's favorite college professor 16 years earlier.

Recalling his warm friendship with Morrie, Mitch regretted losing contact with him, but more important, Mitch realized he had also lost touch with the life-affirming lessons Morrie taught him. Mitch reunited with Morrie and flew from Detroit to Boston every Tuesday to take one last class from the dying man.

Near the end of the book, Mitch asked Morrie a hypothetical question about a promising new ALS treatment in the news. When Mitch asked if Morrie would take a medicine that would reverse his illness to get him back the way he was before he got sick,

Morrie said he would refuse. His illness had forced him to confront the ultimate questions which had to do with love, responsibility, spirituality, and awareness, and for that he was grateful. Morrie had led a full life before the illness, yet something vital was missing that could not be examined until he shifted the flashlight of his attention. People focus on learning about the external world, and what they need to do to be successful there. And physicians are no different. We focus on the external world as we find out what's wrong with the infirm other.

■ TIME AND TERMINALLY ILL PATIENTS

I attended a guest lecture in medical school which reported on the amount of time physicians devote to terminally ill patients. It shrinks dramatically once the patient is deemed terminal. After all, isn't our time best spent with those we can help? Or, does our inability to save the terminally ill patient induce feelings of inadequacy and does the subsequent discomfort drive us away from the bedside? And do our patients need less from us when they are dying?

So, the most educated among us, including physicians and professors, spend most of our energy investigating the world "out there" while ignoring spirituality and the other ultimate questions. That may be OK because spirituality, after all, is someone else's turf. But, as physicians, we have, as a vocational hazard, people in our practices whose world has stopped and are unable to continue doing what had kept them from examining the ultimate questions. Because they may have shared very personal information with us and been more vulnerable than ever before, they may tell us things no other human being has heard including spouse and clergy. Our patients may open their inner door to us, inviting us to go where no one else has entered. Can we refuse? Is it really someone else's job?

What Is Soul?

Our spiritual dimension, the foundation on which humans are built, was clothed with atoms by the sexual union of our parents. They each provided 23 chromosomes to complete the necessary complement for our human vehicle. Although they gave life to physical beings, what about their children's spiritual essence? Plato talked about crossing the river of forgetting when newborns emerge from the womb. Which part of them does the forgetting—and the remembering?

■ A GOD MEMORY

The oldest of our four daughters gave me her definition of soul at an early age. One night, when Hope was 3 years old and we were saying her bedtime prayer, I asked, "Hope, each night we say this prayer: 'Now I lay me down to sleep, I pray the Lord my soul to keep.' What is a soul?" She didn't hesitate a second. "Well, a soul is a God memory." Wow! I was touched. With a tear running down my cheek, I said, "I can't think of a better definition of a soul: a God memory."

Almost twenty years later, I still can't think of a better definition of a human soul. We are seeded by some mystery that exceeds our ability to comprehend it in total. We have some memory of something that draws us to it, some connection to reestablish, some circuitry to rewire to get the juice that can heal a life. Augustine said, "God, you have made us ad te," which means to seek thee.

■ THE WAKE-UP CALL

As adults, the memory of what people truly seek fades, just like their childhood, into the distant past. What has replaced spiritual seeking is the pursuit of the American dream, all consuming until people awaken and see the dream for what it is. Getting sick can be the wake up call. The reality that becomes obvious when awakened from this slumber is both physical and non-physical.

The transient nature of the physical world is then understood in a way that is pressing in its immediacy. The human body is often seen as a vehicle for earth travel, a handy place to hang out and learn about life, but is not required for soul survival. But sooner or later human bodies will provide a lesson in letting go like it or not because eventually people will have to face their mortality. Besides, who would want to stay around in a decaying pile of worm food, to quote Ben Franklin ("Here lies Ben Franklin, food for worms").

There is, also, the non-physical "us" made in the image of God—the child of God that precedes physicality and proceeds without discreet physical morphology upon death. The suffering, chronically ill patient may be more aware of this than most physically healthy folks. The changes in psyche and soma may have forced some hard looks at what was an unexamined life, with the illness serving as the exam that brings the student into contact with life, redefining the significance of living fully. As Morrie Schwartz said, "You can't learn to live until you learn to die." In a culture where the fountain of youth is sought and death denied, most people will learn less about living meaningful lives and more about survival skills, which are important but not enough. People can survive their whole life and never live it. "The unexamined life is not worth living," could be rephrased to: "The unexamined life is not worth surviving." Living fully is what it is all about. Twelve spiritual principles that offer guidance in abundant living for transient earth dwellers will be explored in this book.

The Brain

Because stress occurs throughout the life cycle, healthy coping skills to reduce its impact are so important they should be taught in school. But, they're not. As clinicians, encouraging patients to practice stress management techniques daily helps lower the stress thermostat and ultimately makes them feel better. Patients can gain a better understanding of the brain's role in health and healing by learning about the model of the multidimensional human (MDH) and their triune brain structure. Human brains are composed of three main developmental parts: reptilian, mammalian and the neocortex—the last to develop.

The reptilian brain evolved first and is involved in the automatic regulation of blood pressure, heart rate, appetite and body temperature. The mammalian brain, next to evolve, sits atop the brain stem. The mammalian brain is the limbic system, also known as the emotional or "feeling" brain. The neocortex, the "thinking" brain, is the seat of reason that lies atop the limbic structures and is one-eighth to one-quarter of an inch thick.

Elmer Green, Ph.D., founder of the Voluntary Controls Research Group at the Menninger Foundation, devised his Psychophysiological Principle to describe the connections between these structures. The principle states that for each change in our mental or emotional state, conscious or unconscious, there is a concomitant change in our physiological state. The reverse is also true. For every change in one's physiological state, there is an alteration in the emotional or mental state, conscious or unconscious.

This principle fits with a holistic view of life. According to a fundamental law of nature, everything is connected to everything else. Because people are a part of nature, there are many connections between the cortex and the limbic system, which is well connected to the lower brain centers, the hypothalamus and pituitary gland. People's thoughts (cortical function) drive their feelings (limbic function), causing changes in body and behavior. The wiring is set up for the body to function as a slave to the brain. What people do between their ears reflects itself as physical change at a distance from the brain—even way down in the feet.

■ A HEALING EXPERIENCE: SAVING A FOOT

As a resident in family practice, I met Jim, a patient in diabetic keto-acidosis. I was on call this particular evening when Jim arrived. He was a black, middle-aged man who smelled like acetone. The family had no idea that Jim had diabetes. Upon examination, we found that his left lower extremity was badly infected and gangrene was present. We started an insulin drip, and he eventually woke up. He told us that a couple of weeks earlier, he had cut his foot mowing the lawn, but since it didn't really hurt, he didn't pay much attention to it. His diabetic neuropathy provided dangerous anesthesia, deadening the pain. The infection threw his diabetes into high gear, and he arrived on a stretcher, close to death.

The consulting orthopedic specialists wanted to amputate Jim's foot. Their logic was clear: The patient had a serious infection of the soft tissues as well as osteomyelitis, which required high-powered, intravenous antibiotics to cure. But, you can't get "drug to bug," using the orthopedist's language, because diabetes is among other things, a vascular disease. The impairment of vascular function inhibits IV antibiotic delivery. The solution is to cut off the foot to contain the infection.

Jim did not have a physician when he entered the hospital and became my patient. After I told Jim he had diabetes, I explained the pathophysiology of the disease, including the vascular problem that drove the orthopods to recommend surgical intervention. Believing Jim might be able to save his foot from the surgeon's scalpel, I told him he could learn to vasodilate in the periphery through the use of thermal or temperature biofeedback. He could increase the amount of antibiotics that were being delivered to the area by warming his big toe. The logic was simple. Blood is warm, 98.6°F. If he could warm his toe, he would be not only opening up his blood vessels to carry more blood, but also delivering more drugs to the area through the expanded vessels.

Jim was willing; after all, this was his foot we were trying to save. We began his biofeedback training with hand warming. Learning to warm your hands is facile, a skill anyone can easily learn. Next we transferred the hand-warming technique to his foot, a more difficult task. We gave him a goal of 95°F and taped a paper temperature device to his big toe so he could see the mercury level himself. Motivated to learn because he had something to lose, Jim practiced on his own many times daily.

While the surgeons were skeptical, Jim was diligent. He learned to warm his toe to the goal temperature, and eventually saved his foot from amputation in the process. By learning that he could make a difference, Jim became an empowered patient, who found he could use his mind as a tool to control his body. His cortical control of limbic function not only allowed him to decrease sympathetic tone and allay anxiety, but also to vasodilate and save his foot.

There was something for Jim to learn about himself and his own potential from the presence of diabetes in his life. This story illustrates spirituality in action. Jim gained self-knowledge, learned about his own God giftedness, or how to let go and let God. By applying the passive aspect of our will, or passive volition, we let things happen at their own pace instead of forcing the results. When we pay attention to something, we allow energy to flow in that direction. In the process, we acquire a new way of attending to the present moment and a very practical tool for investing our energy so that we get the best return on our investment. Instead of constantly reacting to external stimuli and allowing circumstances to control our behavior and moods, we switch to an inner locus of control.

Jim also used visual imagery to support his healing efforts, reflecting his belief system of Jesus Christ as the Great Physician. He visualized Christ at the foot of his bed, with light from Christ's healing hands entering his wounds. Though he placed his wounded, sick foot into the care of that Healer, Jim was also participating in his own healing.

When mind, body and spirit work together to heal, they form a powerful synergy. Jim brought his own beliefs into the hospital with him, gladly sharing them with me before putting them to work. He coupled his new learning about the body–mind connection with his own beliefs in a synergistic way. Of course, I'm not diminishing the importance of the medication delivered by IV. It was vital. But, it worked better when the patient actively participated in the healing experience. If Jim could not have participated in his own healing, his anxiety would have been exacerbated. He would have waited, hoped and prayed while the experts took over. Life becomes very stressful anytime someone loses control over their health and becomes passive and dependent on the external medical "fix."

■ WHAT CAN BE LEARNED FROM THE EXPERIENCE?

The question of gnosis, the Greek word for knowing, is addressed at every level of the multidimensional human (MDH). What is there to learn from the illness and its timing? What changes can be made to lead more purposeful and fulfilling lives? All components—physical, mental, emotional, and spiritual—are connected and interdependent, so when people do something healthy for one part, it benefits the whole. A traditional medical model empowers patients with diabetes more than other infirmities. In patient education sessions diabetics learn about their disease, wound management, infection control and how to monitor their blood sugar levels and regulate their insulin intake. They are also taught about diet, how to increase insulin receptors with high fiber intake, and the importance of exercise in stimulating the pancreas to produce more insulin. Some programs are pretty good at stress management, which is very important for people with diabetes because an exaggerated stress response can elevate blood sugar.

So, the top three levels of the multidimensional human—physical, mental, and emotional—are usually addressed in diabetes education programs, but spirituality, the last dimension, usually is not.

■ LOOKING BEYOND THE SYMPTOMS

When I first begin a relationship with patients, I spend 90 minutes asking questions that look beyond their symptom complex to help me view the problem within the context of the patient's life. I ask all sorts of questions that are personal and open-ended, allowing the patients to choose the topics and explore them at their comfort level. In a sense, they tell me their life story, including details about their family and social history. I ask them about their personal and family chemical use, relationships, and what they do for fun. I tell them to pretend I am a genie who pops out of a bottle and will grant them three wishes. What would they wish for that is personal? I'm not looking for answers in the world peace category; I want them to take a risk and reveal more about themselves. It speaks volumes if, for example, one of their wishes is not to be free of the problem that brought them to me in the first place. I ask them to tell me about their religious or spiritual life and their thoughts on the meaning of their illness. If they imagine their life as a movie, how would the illness fit or not fit? I ask them to describe stressful experiences prior to the illness. If a patient confides in me that 18 months ago he cheated on his income tax returns and now thinks his illness is God's punishment, I would explore his thoughts about God. I would ask him to think of characteristics that balance the punitive image, such as the forgiving, merciful side of God. Or perhaps I'd suggest that the patient consider making amends to the government.

There are social taboos warning us not to discuss politics or religion. But, I do not use the term spirituality here to mean a set of beliefs defined by religious dogma; instead it is about how people view and experience their lives and the world with reference to God. You may be thinking that you can't spend 90 minutes interviewing each patient about his or her beliefs, especially if you are in a managed care setting. As a physician, I can appreciate the demands on your time. But, a recent study showed that a patient is allowed to speak an average of only 18 seconds before being interrupted by the doctor. If you were sick and needed medical care, do you think this kind of interaction would be healing? Would you feel you were heard after only 18 seconds?[2]

■ THE 90-MINUTE GROUP OFFICE VISIT

If you feel 90 minutes per patient for an initial appointment is extreme or unrealistic, consider leading a small support group for 90 minutes a day. If you led one group of eight patients a day, four days a week, that would equal 32 patients per week. This will enable participants to discuss what is important to them in a group setting. Discussions often include spiritual matters. After forming the group, you can work on how to create a healthy, respectful environment where people can participate freely.

Strategies for Practicing Holistic Health Care

I suggest that you give assignments to patients, such as journaling, or completing a personal history at home. Then, have them share portions with the group, provided they are comfortable with that. There are limits to what people can risk, so allow them to move at their own pace. As a clinician, would you be willing to share your own story in such a setting? Would you be willing to give them a glimpse of the real you—not just your successes, but your defeats, losses, mistakes, and failures? Would you be willing to reveal your fears? Your willingness to be vulnerable with them helps create a safe environment for risk taking—an unfamiliar role for us in the doctor–patient relationship; we are accustomed to staying safe while our patients take all the risks. I encourage you to experiment with various approaches to discover what works best for you and your patients. Through research and trial and error, science stumbles toward truth. We're scientists, aren't we? Be scientific in your approach toward the exploration of spirituality. Who knows, you may find some truth along the way.

■ ELIMINATING THE EGO

Early in my medical practice, I thought I knew exactly what patients needed to be healthy. After completing a physical exam, I would hand the patient a complete wellness program to follow. I would follow-up a week later and notice that they weren't following the plan. The problem was me—my control issues—not their resolve or initiative, and the solution was to get my ego out of the way. There is an inverse relationship between control and motivation: the more controlling we are, the less likely we are to motivate others.

Connecting the Dots

After a patient's initial visit, it's time to connect the dots. It will create a picture of the patient's illness within the context of his or her own life. If clinicians collected extensive information about the patient's family and social history, they can begin to see how the chronic illness fits into their patient's life story.

The multidimensional human (MDH) is an excellent model to use with patients (Figure 3-1). It can be used as a tool to clear away the brushwood to explore what lies underneath the illness, which is the excuse the person has for taking this journey. Think of human beings as analogous to icebergs. Just as the tip of an iceberg represents around one-tenth of the iceberg's total volume, so too does the physical body represent just a fraction of one's totality. People's behavior, observable by definition, also is part of the tip. People are more than a body acting out behavior sets on the world stage. People are also emotional, mental, and spiritual—these other dimensions are not so easily examined because they exist below the surface of the waters of life.

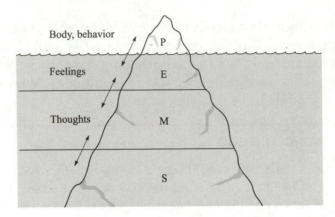

Figure 3-1 The multidimensional human.

The illustration shows how a person's emotional self resides just below the surface. Someone may seem calm, cool and collected on the outside, depending on what they want others to see. The mask may be convincing, while inside they feel anything but calm. "Never let them see you sweat" becomes the normal, but unhealthy slogan. People typically show only their face cards, holding the rest of the hand close to the vest. In some cases, illness results when the body rebels from the incongruence of continually pushing real emotions below the surface.

When people learn to express only what is safe to say and repress the rest, they depress their emotional self. Shakespeare said, "To thine own self be true and thus it follows as the night the day, thou canst be false to any man." Most people don't learn to be true to themselves, and consequently are false to many people.

The mental dimension or thinking self resides below the emotional level. Throughout people's life cycle they need to examine and re-examine the way they think about themselves and the world if they want to lead more authentic lives with depth and meaning.

An illness may provide the opportunity to re-think and re-decide how they see the familiar. It is normal to function on automatic pilot, navigating through the routine of everyday life with all the settings on our habitual patterns. These rote behaviors create a map in the psyche that are traveled because this is what adults in society do. People go to work, pay the mortgage, make car payments, raise the kids, feed the dog, clean the house, do the laundry, serve on differ-ent committees, maintain their bodies, watch TV, go to the kids' activities, go out for dinner, plan for retirement, wonder where the years went, watch their parents decline, work for that promotion, get passed over (unfairly, of course), go on vacation, wonder where Uncle Sam puts all their money, wonder where everyone else gets all their money, wonder where their memory went, read the obitu-aries, and in short, miss the possibilities of the moment.

It is normal to be on automatic pilot, but it does not lead to more expansive lives; people miss things as they look, but do not see. When they are sick, they are in a psychological space where they have a chance to reconnoiter.

Below the mental dimension in the spiritual domain, an inner space from which their thoughts arise. Their thoughts do not usually spring up from the void, but from a set of beliefs, which support their thinking. An old friend, Bob Anderson, a family physician from the Seattle area, is an elder in the work of holistic medicine in general, and more specifically, in exploring this dimension. He says that believing precedes seeing, or that people's beliefs determine what is true for them. The placebo response is an example of the power of people's beliefs to heal the body.

Sometimes patients will discover they need to change their belief system. When a mirror is held up and physicians are allowed to reflect on what patients have told them about their beliefs, they may be surprised to realize that their beliefs are not their own after all, but were inherited from culture including their parents, clergy, and teachers.

Another way of thinking of the spiritual domain is to see it as a social dimension because spiritual values are acted out through human relationships. It has been said that religion in its purest form is love in action; spiritual values have no potency until they affect human interactions.

■ THE JOURNEY IS THE DESTINATION

I take a journey into meaning with my patients that seeks to integrate all facets of being human by helping them learn more about themselves and the role of their illness. The journey inside ourselves is not about arriving at a particular destination; the journey is the destination. Rumi, a 13th century Persian mystic poet who would spontaneously erupt with a poem, wrote:

Keep walking
Though there's no place to get to
Don't try to see through the distances
That's not for human beings
Move within
But not the way fear makes you move.

Go to the well
Move as the Earth and moon move
Circling what they love
Whatever circles comes from the center.

(Translation by Coleman Parks)

Exercises in Stress Reduction

As Rumi wrote, "Move within but not the way fear makes you move." Clinicians go into the inner realm of the patient but not the way fear would have them travel. Fear is the driver of the stress response. People with chronic illness have fears, as others do, but it is possible to act courageously in spite of the fears. Though stress may not have caused their illness, the problem that brought them to the doctor's office may add anxiety to their normal load. Although fear drives the stress response, clinicians can teach patients stress management.

It is helpful for clinicians to create an environment in which patients can learn stress reduction skills. If you don't do so yourself, another in your office can. Have them retreat to a quiet room with comfortable chairs to practice. It is also helpful for patients to have something to help them remember what they talked to their clinicians about during their office visit. Writing notes on a flip chart and sending the sheet home with the patient is a viable idea. This gives the patient a record of their session. It serves as a quick reference tool for the patient. Audio tapes are a good tool too, although I do not record sessions. Privacy and confidentiality must be maintained. Clinicians should experiment to determine what works best for both themselves and their patients.

■ STRESS RELIEVER

Because stress is a frequently used word, it is often assumed that people understand the meaning when it is heard in conversation. People may know when they are stressed out, but they do not have a handle on what to do about it. To help patients identify stressors, I start with a free association exercise by asking them to write down what comes to mind when they hear the word "stress." Their responses are variations on common themes in today's busy world. They bring up stressors at work: boss, deadlines, customers, co-workers, resources, technology, lack of recognition, money, time and the intrusive phone. They also bring up issues at home: kids, spouse, taxes, traffic, balance, ex-spouse, money, in-laws, and housework.

This list is an example of stressors, or causal factors. If you take a systems approach to stress, you will find that there are things that cause us to feel stressed as well as our responses to the stressors. When I ask people in individual or group sessions to tell me how they felt or responded when stressed, they may say they felt angry, tense, frustrated, depressed, or tired. Or they may have eaten too much or too little, slept, experienced insomnia, exercised, drank alcohol, yelled at their kids, talked with someone, or withdrawn from social activities. Some say they had a headache, or back and neck pain. As you can see, the responses are far more negative than positive.

I then let them know that my own knee-jerk response to a stressful event frequently makes a bad situation worse. I tell them that our negative responses are culturally acquired, unhealthy ways we have learned to react to day-to-day stressful events.

Negative responses to stress produce unhealthy consequences. If our work and home lives are stressful, as well as the drive to and from work, it is accurate to say that life in general is stressful. Life is stressful, then we die. It may not be an uplifting thought, but it's accurate because, after all, life is unfair. Because the illnesses that bring patients to see us may represent some unfairness, our challenge is to help them respond in more positive ways.

■ THE CHALLENGE OF SYMPTOM RELIEF

Treating patients with chronic illness allows clinicians the luxury of caring for them over a longer period of time. Typically, our attention is on symptom relief, the focus of the medical training of a physician. A patient presents with symptoms; the history, physical exam and testing reveal the diagnosis; and the ensuing treatment should lead to symptom relief. Symptoms–diagnosis–treatment is the sequence. With chronic illness, symptom relief is primary because a cure may not be in the offing.

But relieving the symptoms, while very important, is not enough. The role of physicians is not just about doing what we were trained to do but about using that as a beginning, a place to make a stand for a more holistic approach to clinical medicine. The premise is that the illness provides an opportunity for learning, and not just in terms of a diagnosis. What is the illness trying to teach the clinician and patient about life? What is there to know, as in gnosis? What changes are appropriate for patients in their daily lives? In this journey, clinicians are headed to a place beyond coping with the status quo and merely increasing the patient's comfort through symptom relief. The journey is about changing, not merely coping, for coping with the status quo is the antithesis of change. Although it may help clinicians handle the problem, it does not delve into the root issues so that patients can reshape their lives. Positive coping strategies are effective tools in turning off the stress response and empowering people to have a measure of control over their mind and bodies, but they can also use them to avoid changing their lives.

■ BIOFEEDBACK AND ITS ROLE IN MEDIATING THE STRESS RESPONSE

Biofeedback can be used as a tool for patients to learn how to turn off the stress response and turn on the relaxation mechanism. No one had to teach humans how to turn on the stress button. After all, it is a survival mechanism hard wired into human animals, just like other animals. In the face of perceived threat, people go into a survival mode, and their body is activated to respond to the threat with extra energy. If they are in a state of chronic stress, which holds true for many chronically ill people, the pump is then primed. The acute stressor gets an even more immediate reaction, which may actually be counter to survival. Through negative responses patients may be reacting in ways that worsen their chronic illness.

Stress management will help both chronic and acute forms of stress. As people manage stress, they continue their work in uncovering what the illness is trying to teach them. In stress management sessions, patients can be taught about their interior engineering and its logic. When the animal part of them goes into survival mode, which is the stress response, predictable changes occur. Blood pressure and heart rate go up, muscle tension increases, and blood is shunted from the skin of the arms and legs into the muscles to prepare them for the extra work of fighting or fleeing, known as the flight or fight response.

As the blood moves out of the skin of the extremities, they cool. A temperature device would demonstrate this. The reverse is also true. When we are relaxing, blood moves out of the muscles where it's no longer needed and returns to warm the skin of the arms and legs. Other changes include platelet clumping. Platelets aggregate to diminish bleeding and improve survivability when the human animal is threatened. If we were wounded on the hunt we would want our blood to clot quickly, thereby decreasing blood loss. Blood sugar also increases to provide extra energy to run or fight when threatened. Hence, people with diabetes can exacerbate blood sugar problems as a result of their negative reactions to stressful stimuli.

Acute stress also affects the immune defense system by briefly activating white blood cell function, decreasing the likelihood of infection if we get scratched, clawed or chewed on the hunt. In the face of chronic stress, however, white blood cell function is decreased. This is secondary to the adrenal cortex releasing corticosteroids.

A new field of medicine called psychoneuroimmunology focuses on the relationships that have been discovered and mapped out in three areas: psychological sets, nervous system, and immune defense system responses. We now know that white blood cells have receptor sites for every neurotransmitter we produce. Why should white cells have receptor sites for neuropeptides and neurohormones unless there is some interaction between them?

Patients always are fascinated to learn how their bodies work. Many have heard about the mind–body connection and get engaged in discovering how their thoughts and feelings can translate into physical changes in their bodies. Once they can see these connections through information-based learning, we can begin experiential learning.

Experience based learning allows patients to put the information they learned into practice. For example, I taught groups of patients with blood pressure problems how to lower their blood pressure through thermal biofeedback. First, they learned to take their own blood pressure. Then, they placed a temperature device on their fingers and learned to warm their hands and then their feet by listening to my relaxation tapes. These patients were performing the work of vasodilators, and were lowering blood pressure by opening the vascular bed in the limbs and decreasing sympathetic tone. Patients also performed these exercises at home, measured blood pressure before and after the biofeedback, and kept records. Eventually, many patients were weaned off blood pressure medications. After a while they didn't have to listen to the tapes because they learned to calm down by recalling how it feels to let go, drawing from an inner remembrance of relaxation instead of relying on the tape or other external stimulation. In a group, I could teach ten people these skills at once, and it also allowed them to support one another and become more open and trusting. Compassion is a healing act when our love touches another suffering human being. It is not just healing for them, but also for us.

It is very simple to teach people relaxation skills with the use of biofeedback.[3] They can learn relaxation skills in other ways: contemplative prayer, meditation, breathing exercises, relaxation tapes, guided imagery, and/or some combination of these. But biofeedback has some advantages because it fits with a learning methodology that is familiar to most of us. We learn through feedback loops. Performance is followed by feedback, adjustments, more feedback, and adjustments, until we finally get it.

Biofeedback, or biological feedback, utilizes the same approach, but the activity occurs inside the body. In the case of thermal or temperature biofeedback, a probe is taped to the palmar surface of one of the fingers to register the current, real time temperature of the skin on that digit. The temperature recorded at the beginning of the session doesn't matter because the goal is the same regardless of where the patient begins. The objective is to increase the initial temperature, and mastery is reached when patients can warm their hands to 96.5°F, or above.

When patients understand the logic of hand warming and the benefit of learning to relax, the rest is a matter of practice. One key point to relay to beginners is that trying too hard is counterproductive. If you try hard to warm your hands, you will stress yourself and your hands will probably cool. You have the intention of warming your hands, but you use another aspect of the will to bring it about. Instead of using the active volition, the active component of the will, you use the passive volition. This passive component of the will is not one fully developed by our cultural training. We learn to use our active volition to make things happen out there in the external world. You decide you want to tear a wall down in your house to make way for an addition, and you try hard, banging away at the wall, until it is down. Voila! Success!

Your passive volition would not be very helpful in that task. Most of what we have accomplished in the world is through active volition. No one has to teach us how to use this aspect of the will because we learned it growing up. Remember as children what we heard from the grown-ups was the secret to success? Hard work! Well, we know how to work hard and try hard, but it isn't useful in learning to relax, to de-stress. So the patient begins to develop a latent aspect of their potential and to pay attention to something dormant. They soon see they can learn self-quieting skills that they can utilize any time, any place. This is empowering because they realize that their efforts can affect how their body works and begin to wonder what else they can do.

I have found that once patients learn to do the training, they can practice on their own. They learn hand warming by listening to relaxation tapes, track their home sessions on a data log, and bring the data to our meetings. I check their data logs and deal with problems or questions fairly quickly. Then, the duration of our session can be focussed on the journey into meaning or to see what there is to learn from the illness as it fits into the story line of their lives.

■ THE BALANCING ACT

When a chronic illness throws patients' lives off balance, we can assist them in restoring equilibrium. I have an exercise that may seem peculiar, but has helped me practice balance. It allows me to use this balance in my everyday life. My friend Patch Adams, the physician on whom the movie of the same name is based, taught me how to walk a slack rope in his back yard. You don't need much equipment. Just a thick, strong rope and two trees or posts that are approximately 20 feet apart. First, you tie a rope between two trees so that when you place all your weight on the rope, it rests just above the ground. You could call that downsizing your risk. Then, you stand next to the rope facing one of the trees. The idea is to place one foot upon the rope and to gradually shift your weight from the ground to the rope. Once all your weight is on the rope, balancing on one foot for the count of five, you've earned the right to take a step. Now, would you think it wise to attempt this new endeavor with your shoes on? Hardly. To get your balance you have to be able to feel the rope. The soles of your shoes would prevent your feet from not only feeling the rope but also gripping it.

Next, place your foot upon the rope and shift your weight to the rope. As soon as you attempt this move and your weight is on the rope, it begins to swing. A slack rope is different than a tight rope.

When you step on a tight rope it begins to move just a little bit, it quivers, but when you step on a slack rope it begins to swing a great deal.

If you feel the rope with your feet and focus your attention where your feet are on the rope, you will quickly fall to the ground since you will be focusing on something that is moving, the swinging rope. The only way to get your balance and stay on the rope is to focus on something that doesn't move. Focus directly on the knot of the rope on the tree trunk straight ahead. By focusing on this immovable object and feeling where you are on the rope, you can achieve your balance. Once you have your balance, count to five—1001, 1002 ... and when you have reach 1005, place the other foot upon the rope and take a step. Sure, you will fall off a number of times learning this new skill. Like all newly acquired skills, you will gain mastery through trial and error. Eventually, you learn to step forward toward the knot, which draws you toward it, and soon you will be walking the rope.

The reason I mention the slack rope example is simple. Remember, the chronically ill have to manage change as a way of life, and slack rope walking is a wonderful metaphor for learning how to do that. Let us look at what the metaphor tells us. First, we need to take off our metaphorical shoes and experience the feelings associated with change, which is better for our overall health than numbing our emotions through denial, medication, alcohol or overworking. Our feelings, the barometer indicating where we are in life, may be trying to teach us something. Acknowledging our feelings brings us into the present moment, instead of rummaging in the past or projecting into the future. Though our feelings are sacred and need to be honored, we also get bogged down in emotions that wax and wane, such as self-pity or victimization. When dealing with the emotional roller coaster that accompanies change, we need a reference point that is constant, like the knot on the tree that provides the focal point for regaining our balance. The 12 spiritual principles I referred to earlier form the strings of the knot, representing values that cannot be changed by our circumstances.

Spiritual Support for Physicians

Are you on a journey to wholeness? Do you feel isolated on the path toward emotional and spiritual maturity? Do you have a spiritual advisor who counsels you along the way, to whom you totally reveal yourself? If not, is there anyone in your life with whom you can be totally vulnerable? If your answers reflect that you are lacking in spiritual development and support, stop right here. Before you begin to mentor you patients in this area, first apply the principles in this book to the man or woman looking back at you in the mirror each morning. Make yourself and your spiritual development the priority. As Rumi said:

> If you are separated from those in spiritual labor
> You are thrown down.
> You are a part without its whole.
> And if the enemy of ecstasy finds anyone cut off
> From that whole
> He experiences him all alone
> And eats him up.
>
> (Translation by Robert Bly)

One of my greatest accomplishments is "owning" my own neediness. We have grown up in a culture where individualism and self-sufficiency are greatly admired. Joseph Campbell, known for his writings on comparative mythology, described the myth of the Grail Quest as the fundamental myth of western culture. Knights went on quests by entering the forest alone, under cover of darkness, in a place without paths. This myth mirrors the cultural notion that we must blaze a trail or follow someone else's, and we must do it alone. Isn't that what our culture reveres? We celebrate people who have achieved success through the strength of their efforts and have pulled themselves up by their own bootstraps. What is so enduring about that expression? Isn't it obvious that our culture resonates at this frequency? We so admire self-sufficiency that we don't ask for help, even when we need it.

When people come to see me for medical care, they honor me by allowing me to participate in their lives in a meaningful way.

When I ask someone else for advice I honor them, and like me, they enjoy making a difference in someone's life. I am now willing to ask for mentoring from fellow travelers on the path, but I am selective about whom I ask for such counsel. Many people do not know how to give healthy support, even people who love us. It isn't that they don't want to support us in a healthy manner; they just don't know how. Most people think they learned how to support others by osmosis from childhood mentors—parents, coaches, clergy, and teachers. They imitate what they learned from the grown-ups, but it may have been unhealthy.

Finding a good spiritual advisor can be difficult, but if you pay attention, you will locate someone with whom you can connect. Be suspect if the person tells you how to move along this path. As a general rule, good spiritual advisors don't tell you what to do, but suggest options to consider. They don't use your failings and missteps in life as an excuse to reinforce your feels of inadequacy, but hold you in an unconditional, positive regard, like a good therapist.

Their support is nurturing, which doesn't mean they always tell you what you want to hear. Because they have done their own inner work, they recognize their human failings and control issues, understanding from their spiritual path how to serve you. They also maintain a connection to a group of seekers to support their own spiritual growth and mentoring of others.

In some spiritual support systems, people submit total control of their lives to another. In the Far East, for example, there is the tradition of the guru–chela relationship in which the student, or chela, relinquishes control to the guru and does not question the authority of the guru on anything. Questioning students find themselves outside the ashram without support. This system's authoritarianism goes against the grain for most individualistic Westerners. Ironically, the control that is supposed to be the glue binding the guru and chela often undermines and destroys the relationship.

If your point of reference is the external, material world, you are always giving your control away to others. It may not be as overt as the guru–chela tradition, but you are giving your power away nonetheless. It's not unhealthy when a student consciously decides to turn his or her power to the guru for some perceived benefit, such as acquiring a higher level of consciousness. A similar situation occurs in A.A. when a recovering alcoholic gives control to a sponsor, who offers counsel and direction. The situation becomes unhealthy when you give power to someone or something and are unaware of it. You have probably known of practicing alcoholics who are ruled by their addiction, but proudly announce they don't really need a drink and could quit tomorrow if they decided they wanted to.

Only you can determine the type of support system that works best for you. Spiritual direction has been very valuable for me on my journey with others. I believe we need spiritual support ourselves before we can mentor others. I suggest that patients also find a spiritual support system, if they don't already have one. The small group process is invaluable for seekers, and Twelve-Step programs are among the many possibilities.

You can find out about spiritual directors in your area through community resources, or by contacting Spiritual Directors International at 1-415-566-1560 or logging onto their website at www.sdiworld.org. Spiritual directors in the network may be members of established religious orders or laypersons. The group publishes a membership directory and a journal on spiritual direction called *Presence*. It doesn't matter how you find someone with whom to share your journey, but for those of us who choose to explore spirituality with our clients, it is important to have our own mentors.

Background Information

Exploring the clinician–patient relationship within a spiritual context puts us on transrational ground, which transcends science and technical reason. Those who believe that it plants us on irrational ground might agree with Sigmund Freud. In his book, *Future of Illusion*,[4] he explores how the world of the religious or spiritual person represents an escape back to the womb. When they are unable to confront the here and now rationally, people escape to a safe place.

Freud felt that reason was the highest human attribute. If we are relying solely on reason, we quickly recognize it is impossible to dissect a human soul out of a cadaver. Therefore, it does not exist. *Homo sapiens* is the end product of evolution, and reason separates us from our primate relatives. With reason we discern two principal drives of the human psyche: love and work. Love here is the sexual impulse that allows the species to survive through procreation.

Despite Freud's pioneering work in the exploration of the human psyche, his view was biased because he denied there is a presence within us that transcends human comprehension. How ironic, since Freud introduced a completely new understanding of human personality by demonstrating the existence and power of the unconscious, by guiding patients in tracing and interpreting their unconscious processes. Psychoanalysis was an attempt to scientifically dissect the human mind and unravel the knotted impediments to healthy, guilt-free sex, and meaningful work. In some ways, Freud was as religious a believer as those on whom he projected his beliefs. His religion was science and his beliefs reflected not a faith-based, but a reason-based cosmology.

Freud collaborated with Swiss psychiatrist Carl Jung from 1906 to 1910, when Jung defected from Freud's group of followers. According to Jung, he and Freud interpreted one another's dreams while crossing the Atlantic Ocean together. Both believed that the unconscious mind delivers messages to us via dreams through symbols. Jung was analyzing one of Freud's dreams when Freud suddenly refused to cooperate, fearing that his answers to Jung's questions would cause the younger psychiatrist to question Freud's authority. At this point, Jung realized his work with Freud was over because Freud was interested more in maintaining his authority and the integrity of his theories than pursuing the truth.

A basic assumption of Freud's theories is that the superego is a censor, a part of the psyche that transforms disturbing and unacceptable thoughts such as the Oedipal conflict into dream symbols. We could not tolerate knowing that we want to have intercourse with the parent of the opposite sex, so the superego creates symbols that are barely comprehensible, but acceptable to our consciousness.

Jung rejected Freud's notion that an unconscious part of us was trying to deceive us. He discovered something entirely new, however, a transrational component of the unconscious that takes us past reason into mystery, which he called "das Selbst," or the self. According to Morton Kelsey, a Jungian therapist and Episcopal priest, this aspect of us seeks to bring us to wholeness whether we desire it or not. For those of the Christian persuasion, Kelsey describes this as the work of the Holy Spirit. Whatever one calls it, I like the idea that part of me is secretly working on my development. I need all the help I can get. Unfortunately, instead of examining our inner lives, we spend most of our time focusing on and reacting to the environment. "If only he had not said that to me, I would not be angry." "If that situation had not occurred, I would not have yelled at my children." "If my spouse would change, everything would be better." These tired scripts are constantly running through our minds, and this is victim thinking. This stimulus–response dynamic is animal consciousness at work because for animals, survival depends on constant surveillance of the environment and rapid reaction time.

The normal modus operandi of humans is to have an external locus of control, just like other animals. Because of this, some psychologists, including B.F. Skinner, have developed psychological models that use environmental control to change behavior. Skinner, the foremost advocate of behaviorism, maintained that conditioning, reinforcement or punishment can shape and define behavior. Skinner defines a human being as behavior in response to the environment. According to Skinner, there is no inner being yearning for freedom and no free will or a soul. We are our behavior, period. I saw Skinner interviewed on a morning talk show when his two-volume autobiography was published. He said, "If what I believe is true of the human condition, the title of my autobiography should be "The Autobiography of a Non-Person." Uplifting, isn't it?

Skinner agreed with Freud that we are animals with reason. If events in the environment drive our behavior, not our thoughts or feelings, then controlling people is as simple as controlling their environment. Sometimes it works, though in a superficial way.

Let me give you an example of how behaviorism works. Let us say you have a young student in whom you are trying to instill a love of reading. You believe that if a child learns to love reading, the world opens up by turning the pages of a book. As positive reinforcement, you give the child a dollar for each book read. Read a book, get a dollar. Another book, another dollar . . . book, dollar . . . book, dollar. Then, the child reads another book and no dollar. "Hey, where's the dollar?" she asks. What did the child learn to love? She loved getting the dollar, but did not change fundamentally. The intrinsic satisfaction that comes from reading was still at a distance from her present life experience, and when the dollars stopped, so did the reading.

Skinner wasn't all wrong. We are programmed, to a certain extent, to perform in proscribed ways to specific stimuli. We all carry culture like a baton that we pass from generation to generation. But instead of thinking that behaviors define us, maybe they are more like garments we wear. We can choose to put on a different garment regardless of what is occurring in the environment. When that happens, we seize our own power and stop playing the role of the victim.

Ironically, learning about empowerment may not happen until someone experiences a chronic illness. We will never know with certainty how we will respond in specific scenarios until they occur in real life. When someone gets sick, they often find interior resources present in abundance. And if they don't, are we prepared to serve as fellow explorers seeking spiritual treasures in the shadows of fear and doubt? Let's examine the principles underlying the Twelve Steps from both the perspective of a medical doctor and a clergyman to discover how to enhance the lives of our patients and ourselves.

REFERENCES

1. Mitch Albom, *Tuesdays with Morrie: An Old Man, A Young Man, and the Last Great Lesson*, Doubleday, New York, 1997.

2. Bob Anderson, M.D., personal communication.
3. "Dr. White's Complete Stress Management Kit," available through BowenWhite.com.
4. Sigmund Freud and James Strachey, *Future of Illusion*, W.W. Norton, New York, 1989.

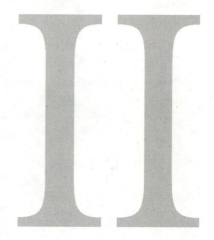

Part II

The Twelve Principles of Spirituality

Chapter Four

Principle 1: Honesty

John A. Mac Dougall

> This above all: to thine own self be true, and it must follow, as the night the day, thou canst not then be false to any man.
>
> Shakespeare, *Hamlet*, Act 1, Scene 3.

> Lead me in your truth, and teach me, for you are the God of my salvation; for you I wait all day long.
>
> Psalm 25:5

> If you continue in my word, you are truly my disciples; and you will know the truth, and the truth will make you free.
>
> John 8:31–32

Step One and the Honesty Principle

Step One states: "We admitted we were powerless over alcohol—that our lives had become unmanageable."

■ THE IMPORTANCE OF HONESTY

The successful treatment of chronic illness calls for rigorous honesty. Clinicians need honesty in telling the truth about what is known, and what isn't known. Patients need honesty to face their illness the way it actually is and to make clear choices about how to treat it and how to live. With honesty, they can know and speak the truth about their lives. With it, they can gain insight and truthfully apply the other spiritual principles to their lives. Without it, spiritual health and growth is impossible. Without it, they aren't dealing with their own lives. Instead, they are manipulating fictional lives and trying to make them look good.

For chronic illness, honesty involves admitting that they are powerless over their bodies, and that their lives have become unmanageable. They would like to exert their will over their bodies, and have them respond. Sometimes bodies do, but not always. Women, with menarche, pregnancy, miscarriages, and menopause, have many occasions to be reminded that they are not in control of their bodies. Men can keep the fantasy of control going longer. This is a mixed blessing. Men commonly get injured in middle age from playing sports as if they were still 18 years old. Without routine information of their bodies' independence from their will, they are free to imagine that if they expect to avoid heart disease, they will.

People do not control their bodies. However, they can influence what happens within them. For example, if they are cold, they can put on a jacket if one is available, turn up the heat if they are inside, drink a cup of warm coffee if it's there, but they cannot will themselves to be less cold. When spring comes and it's bathing suit season, they cannot cause themselves to be more trim. They can diet, and possibly lose weight over time, they can exercise, and gradually convert fat to muscle, they can buy a bathing suit that disguises their flaws, but they cannot choose to have a different body type on the spot.

When people are very young, they don't ''have'' bodies. They ''are'' bodies. Little children run, play, fall down, pick themselves up and go on much easier than adults because their bodies aren't usually giving them very much trouble. Children learn to ski much easier than adults because they aren't as aware of the risk of accidents and they have few experiences of their bodies failing to do what they want. As people age, they gradually have more and more experiences of their bodies not being or doing what they want.

Denial: A Normal Response

Denial is a normal response, and can be helpful for survival. If someone loses his/her job, the family assures them that he will find another. They have no specific evidence that this is true, but it boosts their confidence enough that they will go out and look for another job with some sense of hope. If someone comes home with a diagnosis of cancer, the family assures them that they will get through it fine, even though they cannot know that this is true. People who have a determined spirit and the love and support of family and friends are much more likely to recover than people who hear the news as a death sentence and give up.

■ DENIAL

While I was imagining that I could not possibly write this book, nothing got written. When I denied the possibility of failure and began to imagine how it would feel to have it completed, words came.

Overdone, denial can stand in the way of a successful adaptation to life. If people deny the possibility that people over 50 are more likely to have heart attacks, they may avoid a cholesterol test. If they deny the reality of auto accidents, they may not use their seat belts. People who are on high blood pressure medication often do not comply with their treatment plan because they lack symptoms of chronic illness. They interpret "feeling fine" to mean that they don't need medication. People who live in tick infested areas may pass over the public service announcements about Lyme disease that appear in the newspaper because it makes unpleasant reading. They either don't read or don't remember the early symptoms that could bring effective treatment. Only when their symptoms break through their denial do they seek care. By this time, care comes at a greater cost and is less effective. Anyone who still smokes is practicing denial (and is also probably addicted to nicotine). They either don't believe that they will become ill, or are in denial about how much harm it will bring.

The Anti-Aging Craze

The theory of "what we don't know won't hurt us" is not good health care. People spend huge amounts of money on "anti-aging" creams and potions. They deny that time moves in one direction, from the past towards the future, at a steady rate. Today, an increasing number of men are getting plastic surgery to disguise their age. Even the ads for the American Association of Retired Persons (AARP) show youthful and beautiful 50-year-olds much more frequently than the rate at which they occur in the AARP membership.

At the same time that people deny aging, they disrespect people who are past the midpoint of life. People over 50 have a much harder time getting employed. This is partly due to higher health care costs. A lack of energy and creativity are also suspected. In the computer industry, 40 is considered "over the hill."

■ BLACK BALLOONS

In my workplace, a well qualified professional man got a 50th birthday surprise delivery of black balloons, delivered by a costumed "grim reaper." If this is what his friends think, what chance would he have looking for a new job? The combination of disrespect for older people and denial of aging produces a tension that is hard to talk about openly.

■ THE AVOIDANCE FACTOR

The avoidance of aging is minor compared to the avoidance of illness. I served as a parish pastor for 17 years. Over that time the same pattern was repeated: people who had serious illnesses were isolated from their friends. A diagnosis of cancer would cut most people's friendship groups in half. A common excuse given for not calling or visiting was "I wouldn't know what to say." It was not so much that people made a conscious decision to abandon their friends when ill, but more a matter of avoidance of a painful and difficult subject. Like Scarlett O'Hara in "Gone With the Wind," they said "I'll think about it tomorrow." In the addiction treatment setting, I hear from people who responded to the life threatening illness of someone they loved by getting high. Often, people's addictions get worse as they "treat" the distress of someone else's illness with drugs or alcohol.

I spent 16 years as an emergency medical technician on volunteer rescue squads. In that context, I met many people who denied that they were sick until it became an emergency. Once, I was on an ambulance call in the middle of the night for a man with severe chest pains. It turned out that the man had been having pains for two weeks. He was intending to go to the doctor the very next day. His heart failed entirely shortly after getting to the hospital. Upon being told that the patient had planned to go to the doctor the next day after two weeks of chest pain, the emergency room doctor said, "They can put that on his tombstone!"

The "Nice" versus Truth Factor

Women traditionally have been socialized to believe that being nice is more important than being truthful. Historically, women have been taught to take care of the feelings of others, especially men. Women have also been taught a false modesty that can prevent honest discussions of health and illness. Until 1960, the word "pregnant" was never used on radio or television. It was absent from mass media print, as well. The television show "Laugh-In" broke the taboo with Joanne Worley shouting the word "pregnant" and rolling her eyes, from her perch on the laugh wall. That didn't result in the taboo being broken for everyone.

■ WITHOUT MEDICAL CARE

In the late 1970s an older woman in my wife's church died of advanced metastatic breast cancer. She lived out the natural history of her disease without medical care, because she could not bring herself to use the word "breast."

Admitting Powerlessness over Unmanageable Lives............

Not only are people powerless over illness and aging, but their lives have become unmanageable. This is not as offensive as it might first appear. One slogan is "My life is unmanageable only when I try to manage it." Lives aren't meant to be managed, they are meant to be lived. A Jewish proverb reads: "If you want to make God laugh, tell Him your plans." What happens next cannot be managed. People can respond well or poorly to life's challenges, but they cannot manage them. Alcoholics Anonymous (A.A) speaks of "living life on life's terms." Jesus asked the rhetorical question, "Can any of you by worrying add a single hour to your span of life?" He then advised, "So do not worry about tomorrow, for tomorrow will bring worries of its own. Today's trouble is enough for today." (Matthew 6:27, 34). A struggle for mastery and control only increases stress, not success. "Let go and let God" is a healthier approach to life than "I am the master of my fate and the captain of my soul."

■ **ADAPTING TO CHRONIC ILLNESS**

The beginning of successful adaptation to chronic illness is admitting that we have one. One Sunday after preaching in a church where I was the pastor, I was shaking hands with one of the church trustees. He was an angry, bombastic man. I noticed that he had a bright red blotch in the white portion of his eye. During the coffee hour I pulled him aside and inquired about it. I asked if he had high blood pressure because sometimes a bleed in the eyeball can be a sign of that. He told me it was none of my business and proceeded to launch into a diatribe against doctors and hospitals. I responded somewhat harshly, and asked him how lucky he felt about taking his chances. The next day he went to a doctor and was successfully treated for extremely high blood pressure. On Sunday, he was using anger, denial, blame, and diversion to protect himself from the anxiety

---

of his situation. On Monday, he was more honest and able to seek and receive help. It would be impossible to successfully manage diabetes if we cannot admit having it. Once we honestly admit what's wrong, we also need to admit our need to be part of a network of healing relationships to be as well as possible. We don't heal ourselves. We become well through cooperation with health care professionals, friends, family, and others. Increasingly, people who have similar illnesses are banding together for mutual aid.

A Network of Relationships Are Essential

A.A. is not a "self-help" program. Self-help is a myth. It's a lot like someone tickling themselves. It seems like, conceptually, that someone ought to be able to tickle themself and it should work. But, nothing happens when they try it. They can only be tickled in a relationship. They recover from any illness not by their own will and effort, but in a network of relationships. This includes physicians, nurses, physical therapists, family, friends, counselors, spiritual care providers, and a host of people in roles as simple and important as cab drivers, receptionists, and housekeepers.

In surveys of hospitalized patients, one surprising result is what a great impact friendly housekeepers have on the well-being of patients. Customer surveys often note the positive impact of orderlies and drivers. This network also functions best when there is a trusted Higher Power.

Often, the health care system is a bewildering bureaucracy, even to its employees and professionals. If people envision a Higher Power at work in their midst, and see healing as part of God's plan, they can be more optimistic and confident of a good outcome. Clinicians can use their Higher Power as a source of ultimate values, and as a partner in healing for their patients. Patients can have a Higher Power for comfort and companionship on their journeys.

Honesty is a necessity for all. Instead of trying to be social drinkers, recovering alcoholics admit that they are powerless over alcohol and that their lives have become unmanageable. Instead of trying to be young, they admit their age. Instead of pretending that their health is fine, they do an honest assessment and admit the truth of their situation. Instead of pretending illness will go away, they work with their friends, health care providers, and their Higher Power for wellness.

Not Believing in Death Causes More of It

Part of being well is admitting that everyone is going to die. No matter how vigorous the efforts are for cure, care, and healing, in the long run the mortality rate is 100 percent. The denial of death robs people of life because they then take it for granted.

Teenagers don't really believe that anyone their age dies. This contributes to a pattern of drunken driving deaths. Many years, around high school graduation time, there is a tragic death of one or more students due to drinking and driving. The community is paralyzed by grief for about two weeks. Students swear that life will never be the same now that they understand the fragility of life and the risks of alcohol and cars. Then it blows over, and the behavior of most is unchanged. The pattern repeats on an annual basis. Not believing in death causes more of it.

The denial of death robs life of pleasure. If people deny and avoid awareness of their death, then they act as if they had unlimited time for life. If they have unlimited time, then there is no urgency about anything. They end up wasting time, "killing time", being bored, and neglecting the chance to have passion and adventure in life. It is common for people with a life-threatening illness to have a heightened life awareness. They may derive much more enjoyment from what they do because of the sense that soon they may not get to do it anymore. They declare their love, make amends, savor, and seize the day. People who are sleepwalking through life find little to make it worthwhile.

■ WAL-MART TOASTER THEORY OF LIFE

I have a theory I call the "Wal-Mart Toaster Theory of Life." If you went to Wal-Mart and bought a toaster, and the other person at home asked what it's for, you'd reply, "What do you mean, what's it for? It's obvious from the design. You put bread in the slot, press the lever, and 'toast'. The purpose of a toaster is to make toast." We also come home with a life, one per customer. From its design, we can infer the purpose of life: to be alive. Not just here, not just "not dead yet" but really alive: working, playing, loving and being loved, creating, resting, being silly, experiencing life in all its fullness. One sad outcome for people whose lives are not threatened, is that they are not very alive.

■ SEIZING THE DAY

Chronic illness gives people the license to seize the day and savor it. Frequently coronary care patients say, "I'm glad I had this heart attack. It gives me a new perspective and a reason to drop out of the rat race. I'm going to enjoy my new life." They don't have to wait for a crisis to change their approach to life. They can do it at any point. They need to lay aside their denial of mortality and realize that their lives are perishable commodities. Then they'll be ready to make good decisions about what to do with the rest of their lives.

■ THE SHADOW OF DEATH

One of my friends has just learned that she probably has a recurrence of cancer. She feels well, and the physicians cannot find tumors, but her lab tests show cancer. She's been told to wait until a tumor develops, so that they can treat it. This recurrence brings with it the shadow of death. Instead of living in the shadow, she's bought the houseboat she's always wanted and is enjoying the summer on the Mississippi River. She still makes her medical appointments, but her cancer isn't ruining her life.

Clinicians as well as patients can take hold of this opportunity. There is no reason why the rest of their lives have to be lived under the tyranny of the mistakes and compromises they've made in their lives so far. Looking at their patients can remind them of their own limitations and mortality. Clinicians also need to really live until they die. If they have made unhappy compromises in their honesty, they can recover it. If they have signed HMO contracts with "gag clauses" that make them agents of a distant bureaucracy instead of scientists, healers, and artists, they can let those restrictions quietly expire, and regain their freedom and dignity.

The spiritual principle of honesty provides a way for people to be true to themselves, others, and to the highest possibilities that life offers them, as clinicians, as patients, and as children of God. It is also a way to help their patients be truthful about their illnesses.

Suggestions for honesty in your life and work:

- Admit to yourself that you are powerless to control the outcomes of your clinical practice. You can control what you do, but not its outcome.
- Be honest about the details of clinical practice. This includes appointment times, your own boundaries around time and access, likely effects, side effects, benefits, and risks of proposed treatment.
- Avoid minimizing problems or saying things will be all right when you do not know that to be true.
- Invite your patients to be entirely honest with you, and assure them that if they state unpleasant thoughts or feelings, that will not change your level of care for them.
- Be honest in your financial practices. This includes billing methods, how you compensate employees or partners.

Bowen F. White

There are some values that are basic to living in human relation-ships. They are so obvious, people take them for granted. Honesty is one of those principles. Many people have heard the phrase, "Honesty is the best policy" and probably believe it. But, do they really practice it in everyday life? An initial response most likely is that they are honest. Although they can probably think of plenty of dishonest people, they most likely believe that they are not like them. There are even times when people might be dishon-est without even telling a lie. We often deceive people through silence, a nod of the head, or a wink of the eye.

Honesty takes courage. When confronted with a chronic ill-ness, the risks involved in being honest don't appear as daunting. Honesty becomes paramount. Often, the chronically ill patient comes to the realization that they have no time to waste on being dishonest. When a clinician treats a chronically ill patient, it's time for them to realize that they don't have all the answers when dealing with a chronic illness. Providing a fix for the chronic ail-ment isn't like dealing with an acute illness. There are no easy answers. But honesty is a good place to start. The clinician should start by being honest with themselves. Clinicians should work to establish a rapport with their patients that encourages the principle of honesty. Trust is developed as a result.

■ WHAT HONESTY CAN DO

The consequences of being honest can have some startling results. For example, one of my patients in her mid-thirties was diagnosed with ovarian cancer. She was a nurse who understood what it would take to beat the odds. She was in a failing marriage with two children. The diagnosis of the chronic illness—cancer, gave her new strength. She suddenly felt more freedom than ever before. She didn't care what her husband thought. She was going to live the life she always wanted but was afraid to ask for before the diagnosis. Her unhealthy home environment suddenly became unacceptable as this wasn't the type of life she would ever choose.

For the first time, she began to speak up and started saying what she really thought. Her husband grew more and more aggressive and abusive as his wife started her new way of life. Instead of withdrawing, she started taking risks that before she would never have dreamed of. Despite her chronic illness, she gained self-esteem. She quit putting herself down. As her cancer progressed, she struggled more and more with the issue of leaving her husband. But, she finally made a decision. She did what was healthy for her, what was honest, and what was real for her. She left him. Today, her cancer has been in remission for over 10 years. She has a great relationship with her two sons. Her chronic illness allowed her to quit being an enabler and start to do what she needed to do, what was real, true. The truth set her free. She decided that if she was to die, she wanted to live the rest of her life in a way that was authentic for her and no longer pretend.

I was totally humbled by her courage. As her clinician, I was supportive of what she wanted to do. That type of support was crucial. I didn't tell her what or what not to do. Instead I asked the question, "What can I do to be helpful?" This is acting in an honest and open way.

Adults typically tell children that honesty is the best policy. But, what happened when those children did something they weren't supposed to do and were honest about it? They were punished. As a result, what did they learn to do in order to survive? They lied. They soon discovered that stretching the truth was something adults did on a regular basis without much consequence.

The following example illustrates how children first learned about the consequences of honesty:

> Junior comes home from school. He then walks into the silent living room where his dad is sitting in a chair with his head cradled in his hands. His dad is slowly shaking his head and rubbing his temples with fingers moving in circular patterns.

His eyes are closed. Junior stops abruptly. Although his dad is silent, his body language speaks loudly. Junior moves slowly toward the slumping figure. "Gee dad, what's wrong?" Dad responds, "Nothing." In reality, everything was wrong. He just had a major feud with his boss and walked off the job. Why did he respond by saying, "Nothing"? He learned this behavior from his father. The baton was passed from father to son. What are the justifications that his father used to rationalize his distance from the truth? They are revealed in statements like: "He wouldn't understand." or "I don't want to worry the boy." or "He couldn't help me anyway." He may not have made any conscious decision to deceive his son. His programming by acculturation is to not appear weak. He thinks he's protecting his son by hiding the truth. But, the father can't hide what his body has revealed. So his son knows that his father is not telling the truth. His father's inability to be vulnerable becomes instructive. Dad is leading by example.

Parents often talk about how difficult it is to deal with teenagers. A conversation with Junior may go something like this in the future. "How's it going, son?" "Fine." "Any problems?" "Nope." And shortly thereafter dad discovers that Junior has gotten someone pregnant, is flunking out of school and is chemically dependent. When he inquires into his son's reasons for deceiving him, he may hear, "I didn't want to worry you, dad." or, "I didn't think you'd understand."

Junior has been well schooled by his father. He's doing what he learned. But, it's not just his dad who is demonstrating this communication style. His mom is guilty too. She goes off to church to help prepare a special dinner. When she returns home she says, "I'm never going to help prepare a meal there again as long as Sylvia Jones is in charge. I know it's not very Christian, but it's the truth. I just can't stand that woman."

Six weeks later the family is sitting around the dinner table when the phone rings. It's Sylvia asking if mom can help with the church supper. She ends up saying she'd love to help. As she hangs up the phone, she mutters, "What have I got myself into?" When asked about the obvious incongruity between talk and actions, mom explains, "Although Sylvia drives me crazy, I couldn't say no to her. It would be like saying no to the church. Okay, I wouldn't love to help. It's a lie. But, it's a white lie. And nobody is harmed."

Most people learned about honesty at a young age. Growing up, children all witnessed multiple examples of adult dishonesty. It wasn't just their parents or parental figures. It was ubiquitous adult behavior. Children watched and absorbed. There were always good reasons for the deceit. "I didn't want to hurt her feelings" or "If I were honest about my real opinion I might look stupid in that meeting." It was rationalized by the adults and learned by the children. These children have now grown up. And dishonesty is not someone else's issue. It is everybodys.

■ DISHONEST SURVIVING

As a child, I had to be dishonest in order to survive. If my parents found out about all the stuff I was actually doing, it would have been counter to survival. I was the third of six kids with an over achieving older brother and sister ahead of me. They were star students, musically talented, involved in leadership activities, and well liked. I compared myself to them and didn't quite measure up. I had a different role in the family system. The only reason I knew the school principal well was not through scholastic, musical, dramatic or student congress achievement. Rather, the school principal and I became well acquainted because my teachers sent me there.

I was often in trouble. I ran with the wrong crowd. I did many things that I never wanted my parents to discover. As a child, I was dishonest of necessity. As I grew older, I thought I had outgrown my dishonest ways. Not so. I could not do it alone. One of the books that helped me was *Invitation to a Great Experiment*.[1] The book was originally published in 1959 as *First Questions on the Life of the Spirit*. It showed me ways of developing a more authentic relationship with God. By reading this book and by searching out other spiritual seekers, I discovered that I was honest with certain people and dishonest with others. Deception was my game. I could deceive without ever telling a lie. In reality, I was a very skilled liar.

Today as a conference presenter, I commonly request that "all the dishonest people in the room stand up." Rarely does anyone else rise to their feet. Why don't others stand? They are in denial. We all think of ourselves as honest folks. Unless, of course, your life has turned in such a way that you have overcome your denial and accepted the truth. The irony is this: you can't do anything to become more honest until you accept your dishonesty. Self acceptance is the beginning of change.

Initiation into the healing profession came with a cost for clinicians. Clinicians paid a price to become the experts on what is wrong with other people. Their own dysfunction remained unexplored as they deciphered the esoteric signs and symptoms of the infirm other.

There is no time like the present for clinicians to examine their dishonesty. It is never too late to join the fray with the rest of humanity. Clinicians can begin their own journey toward healing, wholeness, and emotional maturity. That journey begins by overcoming their own denial and accepting the truth about themselves.

■ HONESTY AND RELIGIOUS TRADITIONS

And as a spiritual principle, honesty is a knot that is unchanging and never untied in all religious traditions, regardless of cost. A friend of mine, Don Campbell told me a story about the risks involved with honesty. In the time that preceded our entry into World War II, there were missionaries in China. A group of missionaries were fleeing Japanese invaders. The missionaries were going from town to town on their escape route from China. As the soldiers reached the town where the missionaries were resting up prior to continuing their retreat, a family was kind enough to put them in the upstairs of their own home. The soldiers began searching the town, door to door. Inside their homes, villagers could hear the sounds of boots marching, stopping, marching to the next house, stopping, as the soldiers sought out their prey. Eventually, those sounds signaled the arrival of the death squad at the sympathetic family's door. KNOCK. KNOCK. KNOCK. "Open the door!" the soldiers shouted.

The father of the Chinese family obeyed the soldier and opened the door. "Are the missionaries in there?" the soldier demanded. "Yes, they are," the father replied. "Where are they?" the soldier asked again with authority. "Upstairs," the father replied honestly. "What are they doing?" the soldier asked again. "Praying," the father replied. There was a long pause and then, in a booming voice, "March on!" the soldier commanded. The soldiers left the missionaries to their prayers.

Why didn't the father just lie to the soldiers? He put his own family at risk by his actions. And I would assume that most of us would have lied in similar circumstances. But, we really don't know what we would have done. For us, it is only hypothetical. And the truth cannot penetrate a hypothetical situation. But, the above certainly speaks to the risks involved in being truthful. The risks we face daily would be much less dramatic, we have much less to lose, but we, or at least I, do not have to look very hard to see how I fall short of the honesty policy. How about you?

■ ENERGY FOLLOWS ATTENTION

Energy follows attention. If I pay attention to how I communicate, I then have the energy focused where it needs to be, on me. This may go against what people have been taught in communication seminars for years. When I ask people what was the most important thing they learned, the answer is always the same. "Listening, we need to be better listeners." Indeed. Studies have shown that physicians interrupt their patients, on average, within 18 seconds of their initial words.[2] Now, I don't want to downplay the importance of listening. It is vitally important that we be good listeners. We need to open all three of our ears, the two in our head and the one in our hEARt. While establishing a strong clinician–patient relationship, it is important to realize that people need to feel heard. When the ear in the hEARt is open, people can feel our listening.

But, if you're listening to someone, a patient, your spouse, your child, a nurse, or someone else and that someone is not telling you the truth, is this real communication? If someone is actively attending to something that you are saying but your words lack veracity, is this good communication? Sure, we need to be good listeners. Communication involves sending and receiving. We need to listen to receive what is being sent. But, that is secondary. What is primary? What is primary, what is most important, is that what is being sent is the truth.

The truth will set you free. It will free you to be real and authentic. If you don't know the answers, you will feel free to admit it and ask for help. The Truth is the first and last, the Alpha and Omega that the spiritual journey is about. Honesty can be seen as a pick to clear away the debris from the treasure. It is not the only tool. But you cannot make much progress without it. It's the real thing. Accept no substitutes.

Ways in which you can risk being honest both in your family life and in your relationships with your chronically ill patients might include:

- Our training is all about knowing what is best for others. But, we don't always know what is best for our chronically ill patients. Instead we must listen and give suggestions when asked and admit we don't know all the answers.
- Take time to listen to your patients. Do not interrupt your patients when they are speaking. Listen with your hEARt, the ear in the chest.
- Support your patients in the decisions that they make even if they choose something other than what you would have chosen for them.
- Above all, be honest. Pay attention to how you communicate. Dishonesty is not someone else's issue. Honesty is crucial.

REFERENCES

1. Thomas E. Powers, *Invitation to a Great Experiment: Exploring the Possibility that God Can Be Known*, East Ridge Press, East Ridge, NY, 1986.
2. Howard B. Beckman and Richard M. Frankel, "The Effect of Physician Behavior on the Collection of Data," *Annals of Internal Medicine* 101 (1984) 692–696.

Chapter Five

Principle 2: Hope

John A. Mac Dougall

Hope deferred makes the heart sick, but a desire fulfilled is a tree of life.

Proverbs 13:12

And now, O Lord, what do I wait for? My hope is in you.

Psalm 39:7

Step Two and the Principle of Hope

Step Two states: "Came to believe that a power greater than ourselves could restore us to sanity."

■ ACHIEVING HOPE WITH THE HELP FROM OTHERS

If all a chronically ill patient has is honesty and their own resources, their chronic illness could lead to despair. If the patient has accurate knowledge of their chronic illness, and faces that knowledge squarely, they may despair. If cure seems unlikely, and the patient is limited to their own resources and the help of people who can't cure them, they may gradually withdraw from life. If, however, the patient looks to the future with a sense of possibility, and draws on strength from a power or powers greater than themselves, hope will result. They can come to believe that a power greater than themselves could restore them.

■ SUCCESSFUL ADAPTATION TO CHRONIC ILLNESS

I have had chronic pain from migraine headaches for the last forty years. From 1959 to 1989, I did the wrong thing for them, taking addictive pain killers and tranquilizers, along with alcohol, as my pain management plan. From 1977 to 1989, there was a thought in the back of my mind: "Make friends with your pain, it's part of you." This made no apparent sense, but it was the voice of my Higher Power. It was trying to teach me acceptance and to lead me to a successful adaptation to the chronic illness.

As mentioned previously, a Higher Power can be anything that is: (1) not me, (2) more powerful than me, and (3) wants to help me. This can be a group of people, a spiritual program, Twelve Step group, church, or chronic illness support group. This can be a program of recovery, a philosophy, a sense of unity with humankind, or a religion. It can be an intangible Higher Power, such as God, Buddha, Allah, or a variety of other names or titles. If the patient is on his own, hope is hard to achieve. If the patient is living in a committed community and guided by a Higher Power, hope comes naturally.

Making Peace

A prerequisite for hope is for people to make peace with themselves, and with their chronic illnesses. Successful adaptation is needed not only to the chronic illness itself, but also to the special challenges of daily living that come as a result of the illness. Diabetics must follow a diet and travel with their medications and blood testing materials. Patients who cannot walk can get mobility equipment and plan their travel well. The cancer patient may need to time major life events so that they are not debilitated by the side effects of chemotherapy. Adaptation gives them hope that life can become manageable.

■ ACCEPTANCE

Alcoholics Anonymous (A.A) says: "Acceptance is the answer to all my problems today. When I am disturbed, it is because I find some person, place, or thing unacceptable to me, and I can find no serenity until I accept that person, place, thing, or situation as being exactly the way it is supposed to be at this moment."[1]

Embracing Emptiness

The more patients try to make pain stop, the worse it gets. The more they pretend they don't have pain, the more intrusive it becomes. If, on the other hand, they accept the reality of pain and stop guarding against pain, it may wash over them. However, if they then relax and don't struggle, it begins to recede.

Acceptance does not mean approval, it means the acceptance of reality. They don't have to approve their chronic illnesses. They just have to accept that they are real.

Part of making friends with their pain is to embrace their emptiness. Once they admit their powerlessness, the emptiness of that experience can mellow into a spaciousness, into which hope can come. As long as they are trying to exert power they don't have, life will be characterized by struggle and disappointment.

> ■ **CREATING A SPACE FOR HELP**
>
> Once I admitted that the drug cocktails weren't working, and that I was just drugged and in pain instead of sober and in pain, I created a space for other help.

The Importance of Sharing

As long as patients tell the people who love them that everything's fine, they are cut off from their support. By sharing their hurt, they invite the love of others, as well as their practical help.

There is a process of recovery that begins with finding hope. Members of Twelve Step programs practice their Step Two: "We came to believe that a power greater than ourselves could restore us to sanity." This process is sometimes summarized as "We came, we came to, and we came to believe." These three parts can be understood as presence, awareness, and faith.

Those with chronic illnesses must become present to other people. They will not recover from a chronic illness alone. Human beings are interdependent for almost everything. Most do not grow their own food, weave their own clothing, build their own homes, and distill their own gasoline. People are reliant on others for most of their routine needs. Considering this, it is odd that people often react to a crisis by trying to handle it alone. Chronically ill patients must come into contact and fellowship with others to be well. In isolation they become only worse. To be willing to be in contact and fellowship with others, people may have to answer the "why me?" question.

System theory holds that a pattern of events is not causality. Just because the sun went down after dinner doesn't mean that the sun went down *because* of dinner. When things are going well, people don't automatically suspect that a Higher Power is blessing them, but when things are going poorly, they tend to suspect that a Higher Power is giving them their problems.

■ **"HE LOOKS HEALTHY, LET'S BREAK HIS LEGS."**

I disagree with the statement "God never gives you more than you can handle." The reason I find that disagreeable is that it sounds as if God sits behind a counter and hands out bad things. "Oh, he looks healthy, let's break his legs." "Her life is going well, let's give her cancer. She can handle that." "He's secure, let's give him a mugging." It makes God the author of misfortune and evil.

Randomness, Error, and Evil

Randomness, error, and evil are three sources that aren't always liked. An electric plant uses dirty coal and a thousand miles away three people get sick. Who are these three people? It may be random. A driver falls asleep at the wheel and crashes into someone else. It's an error. Someone chooses to rape and murder because it feels good. That's evil. All three exist. Any belief system that doesn't include randomness, error, and evil, is prone to disillusionment. There is little convincing evidence that God steps in to prevent randomness, error, and evil. Ask the Jews. If God was going to intervene, Hitler would have provided a good occasion, but millions died in World War II. The experience of history shows that randomness, error, and evil hold sway without interference.

The Importance of the Support of Others

In contrast, the experience of millions of men and women in A.A., Narcotics Anonymous (N.A.), Al-Anon, and other Twelve Step groups is that, when it was time to recover, a gracious Higher Power gave timely assistance. So, if their Higher Power doesn't interfere with bad things, but does help with good things in recovery, a sensible response is to minimize their exposure to randomness, error, and evil. People wear seat belts, drink clean water, get regular checkups, watch their blood pressure and cholesterol. They avoid high crime areas and watch their personal security. That's reasonable, but for real change they also need to maximize their exposure to the activity of a loving Higher Power in a program of recovery.

There are many situations in which exposure to the care of other people is helpful in dealing with their problems. Migraine patients commonly get very short doctor visits, followed by a prescription for one drug for prevention and another to treat headaches. The chances are only fair that the first prescriptions will be the right ones, because so many variables are at work. The physician is often under the constraints of limited reimbursement from managed care, and limited medication choices within the managed care companies' formularies. The patient must be dealt with quickly and is unlikely to get the emotional support needed to confront an illness with so many uncertainties. The patient is likely to get that emotional support in a headache support group, such as those offered through the National Headache Foundation. The information received there may be less accurate than from a specialist, but the emotional support, as well as stories of hope and recovery are there.

Gratitude

After natural disasters, when the television crews interview people in front of their wrecked homes, there are often expressions of gratitude for the help of friends, neighbors, strangers, and life itself. Although the disaster is a random bad thing, people who expose themselves to help from the wider community of humankind have good experiences.

■ NO RIGHT ANSWER

There may not be a satisfactory answer when patients or clients ask the "Why me" question. The answer may well be randomness, error, or evil. However, the question still needs to be posed and possible answers at least considered. When people ask, "Why me?" the universe's response may be "Why not you?" Nobody is exempt.

The Importance of a Support Group

System theory also includes the law of entropy, that energy becomes unavailable in a closed system. This is commonly experienced as the tendency of things to "run out of gas." This is true of automobiles, which run out of gas unless more fuel is introduced, and is also true of support groups. They too will "run out of gas" unless there are newcomers joining the group with fresh problems, and new ideas. Then the group can address the problems presented. In this setting, group members come out of isolation into fellowship with other people in recovery. The addict goes to N.A. while the heart attack patient bands together with others in the same situation in a cardiac rehabilitation group. The grieving parent goes to a Hospice support group. In a closed system of self and isolation, nothing new comes in, a downward spiral occurs, and people die as a result.

The most obvious example of a closed system is a person who does not eat. Without energy from outside, entropy sets in and they starve. Babies who have "touch hunger" are diagnosed with "failure to thrive." They aren't thriving because they are alone too much. The alcoholic who tries to control drinking alone gradually has less and less energy available for the struggle to stay sober. Without the "open system" of help from others in recovery, relapse is natural.

System theory states that the whole is different than the sum of the parts (This is often misquoted as "the whole is greater than the sum of its parts."). A.A. brought together a collection of men and women. As individual "parts" none could stay sober. When they banded together they could remain sober. A whole had been created that was far more powerful than a collection of individual alcoholics. The whole is different than the sum of its parts according to the principles by which it is organized. Twenty alcoholics sitting in a bar, with a common purpose of drinking while watching the Super Bowl will be less than the sum of their parts. They may erupt in a fight and be unable to complete their chosen task of drinking. Twenty alcoholics gathered with the outside input of program literature, traditions, and a Higher Power may do great things for and with each other.

Having persevered in joining together for a common purpose, people "come to" and become aware of the hopeful possibilities of fellowship with others. By banding together with others experiencing a similar situation, the hope in their lives is revealed, and they become hopeful. The patient who needs a bypass hears the success of others and has hope. The family of an Alzheimer's patient hears how other families cope and have hope that they may be able to cope with their loved one's needs. Cancer centers offer support groups knowing that their outcomes are better when they do.

■ **CHAPLAIN VISITS**

Back in 1972, when I was in chaplain training at Bellevue Hospital in New York, the city hospitals routinely scheduled chaplain visits with pre-operative patients, whether or not they had a religion. The city government didn't do this to evangelize, but did it because the outcomes of surgery were better when they did.

Gotta Have Faith

Patients need to come to believe in a power greater than themselves. If patients visualize themselves as being on their own, their resources may be too limited for them to thrive. Taking this into consideration, clinicians should inquire into the nature of their patients' beliefs. Questions such as, "Do you have a Higher Power? Is it a god figure, your family, the hospital, a recovery program, a group of friends?" are all appropriate. Having had this discussion, the clinician can invite patients to visualize themselves being cared for by this Higher Power. If the patients' belief systems include prayer, the clinician may choose to offer to pray with or for the patient. Regardless, at the minimum, this should have a calming effect on the patient. Chances are, it may become much more. The hospitalized patient who rings the buzzer and waits a long time for a response wonders if anyone cares. Another patient who knows that the staff is praying for and with her is much more likely to have confidence in the hospital process.

Hope is Power

If patients and clients are powerless over their illnesses, and there is no hope, they are finished. They begin to feel trapped because they either have no Higher Power, or have one that is distant or hostile. Historically, people who have lacked power over the centuries have turned to hope for solace. The people of Israel who had been slaves in Egypt set out on an improbable journey because of hope of a promised land. African slaves imported to the Americas held to hope in order to achieve freedom. Patients who lack power over their illnesses can find solace in hope as well.

In truth, women may turn more easily to hope than men. Any woman who bears a child is embarking on an exercise in hope. Women have been socialized as the nurturers and comforters, and thus have hope as their natural style. Men are more free to imagine that their powers are unlimited, and crash when they meet obstacles. Women are more likely to know adversity and limitations on their power, and to be well practiced in responding to it with hope.

A Channel for Hope

God's name and address are not needed to develop hope, but people simply need an openness to asking for and receiving help. A.A. suggests that the alcoholic ask: "Do I now believe, or am I even willing to believe, that there is a Power greater than myself?" Even the willingness to believe is sufficient, because it can move people forward in their inquiries.

An assessment of spiritual state may help. If people have a religion, is it helping them achieve good relationships with a Higher Power, with themselves, and with other people? If it is a divisive religion, which leads to splits in families and friendships, then it may not be healing them. If it is a religion of coercion and obedience, then it may not be leading them to the freedom of a full life. However, if the religion is characterized by love and service, then they will become more sane and more whole by continuing in it.

People can assess their Higher Powers. They all have powers that are greater than themselves, but those powers may not be healing. People can, through their resentments, have someone become a "Higher Power" who is actually destructive to them. When people resent someone, it's often for a good reason. It may feel as if their resentment is aimed at the other person, but the negative impact is actually on the one who has the resentment. Keeping resentments is like drinking poison and expecting the other person to die. People can have a vengeful ex-spouse as a Higher Power in that the ex-spouse governs thoughts and feelings. One patient identified American Express as his Higher Power. It was the only force he respected because they would cut off his charge card if he didn't pay. People can have an employer as their Higher Power, giving their best at work and leaving the leftovers for family and friends. It is possible to have positive Higher Powers other than God. People can have program sponsors or mentors, groups with whom they have a common cause, positive role models in society, a favorite ancestor.

As people come to believe, fear will be replaced with trust. If they are on their own, they have a lot to be afraid of. Instead, they begin to trust that people in their group are for them. They begin to "trust the process" of recovery. They stop assuming that everyone is out for themselves, and look for people who will cooperate with them. They begin to replace self-pity with gratitude, despair with joy, defiance with surrender, dishonesty with honesty, grief with comfort, and resentment with acceptance.

The Tools of Spiritual Growth

People don't have to have a god-concept at all to begin using the tools of spiritual growth. They can begin to read the wisdom literature of different religions. They can pray, even without knowing to whom they are praying. They can ask for help with their chronic illness or persistent issue. If they do this at the beginning of the day, when the issue comes up they can turn to that unknown Higher Power for help again. At the end of the day, they try giving thanks, even if they don't know who they are thanking or what they are thanking them for. Then they evaluate how life is going after a few weeks of this practice. Even if there was no God, and they were only praying to the best part of themselves, they might get good results.

Once people have been honest with themselves and their situations, and have found hope for a good life, they need to make decisions that support recovery. They make a decision to move forward with faith.

Suggestions for hope in your life and work:

- Come to believe that a power greater than yourself can guide your clinical practice.
- Consider your own hope for your clinical practice. What do you hope for in your personal and professional development?
- Consider first what gives you hope with each patient. What outcome do you hope for with each patient? (This does not have to be the same as the patient's hope, but it is a starting point.)
- Ask each patient what they hope for, with an open ended question. It might be cure, remission, a certain span of life, freedom from pain, a good death, or another hope. Be open to joining them in hoping for their goal.
- Avoid false hope or enforced cheerfulness. Also avoid stating certainties that you don't actually have.

Bowen F. White

Hope is essential as a spiritual principle. Amidst the pain and suffering and unfairness of the world, it is unchanging in its importance. Clearly, it is knot material. Vaclav Havel, a Czech writer and the first president of the Czech Republic, says hope is definitely not optimism. It is not that everything is going to work out all right. But, it is the certainty that regardless of how things work out, one can find meaning in them.

■ THE HIDDEN MEANING

The premise I share with my patients is that the problem that brought us together has meaning/meanings. Regardless of the severity of the problem, there is always hope. Instead of the patient asking "Why me?," how about "Why not me?" Encourage the chronically ill patient to learn something from this life experience. Don't get me wrong, "why me?" is a legitimate question. But, "why anyone?" is just as good. There are things we can't know with certainty as we travel through life. Bad things do happen to good people. It is reality. But "why me?" as a mantra can turn into "poor me." Victim thinking and self pity are unempowering to people. They also eat or drain energy out of our systems at a time when we need to conserve energy to then invest in productive activity.

My patient with ovarian cancer made a decision to leave the life she was living and start a new one in spite of the chronic illness. She left her abusive marriage after recognizing that she needed to take care of herself first. She began to nurture herself and the end result was positive. Of course, not all patients will experience such a remarkable recovery. But, she envisioned hope for a life worth living and she went for it. Others can learn from her example.

The Hopeful Rat

Work done with rats demonstrates the practical benefit of being hopeful.[2] One experiment involves two genetically identical rats, in identical cages, with identical wires around their tails. The wires deliver a bolus of electricity simultaneously into the rats' tails. The electrical shocks are delivered at random. There is no pattern to the unfairness that they experience. One rat (the empowered rat), has a bar in his cage that is hooked up to the electrical device. When this rat presses the bar it turns off the shock for himself and his buddy. The other rat (the unempowered rat), is identical to the first rat and has the same kind of set-up in his cage. There is an identical bar present which he can press, but, it is not hooked up to the electrical device. So, no matter what he does, he cannot turn off the shock. Instead, he has to wait for his empowered friend to press the bar in the other cage to get some relief.

The rats are then shocked at random for three weeks. The empowered rat hangs out in his abode and suddenly gets a shock. He has learned through trial and error that pressing the bar turns off the shock. So, he runs over and presses the bar and experiences relief. His unempowered buddy likewise, hangs out in his cage when zap, he receives the bolus of electricity. He jumps up into the air and runs away from the locale where he was shocked. But is it safe? No, a geographic displacement provides no relief. This is because the wire is around his tail. Wherever he goes, he takes his tail with him. Hence, there is no safe place. If you are wondering about the bar, remember that in his cage it is not connected to the source of discomfort. He already learned it's of no use. And, in fact learned that no matter what he does, it doesn't make any difference. The shock starts by some mystery and stops by some mystery. There is no logic to discern.

The experiment continues for three weeks. At its conclusion, the rats are removed from their cages and placed in water. The empowered rat swims around, looking for the shore or high ground. He has learned that by virtue of his efforts he can effect his destiny. Isn't that what empowerment is about? The unempowered rat does not swim around in the water. Why? He has learned that it doesn't matter what he does, it doesn't make any difference at all. So, he doesn't bother to swim because he feels it wouldn't help him escape the inevitable. That's one depressed rat! He just treads water and is retrieved before he drowns.

Upon the experiment's conclusion, the rats are examined. The empowered rat is healthy while the unempowered, depressed rat has ulcers. It is interesting because they are genetically identical rats who were given the same amount of electrical shock, for the same length of time. Yet one is healthy and one is sick. What was the difference? They both were shocked simultaneously. Yet, one stayed healthy in a very sick environment. Sure, he could turn off the shock. But, did it keep it from happening again? No! The shocking occurred at random. Nonetheless, he stayed healthy.

What was the difference between the two rats? Control. One had control while the other did not. Was the control occurring at the level of input? No, in fact the rats had no control over the fact that life was shocking them. Control occurred at the level of response to input at least for the empowered rat, who could stop the shocking experience temporarily. And, although the shock stopped simultaneously for the unempowered rat, the stress of having no control over his situation was such that he developed ulcers.

Any time people feel as if they have no control over what is going on, it is exceedingly stressful. People have no control over what life puts into their in-box. But, they do have control over how they respond. But many of their learned responses have been to make a bad situation worse by what goes out of their out-box. Then they use that negative response as another reason to feel bad about themselves. It is amazing how unrelenting they can be in their abuse of themselves. They do not even need the world to shock them. People are experts at this work. The following example illustrates this point nicely:

> The expressions "Yeah, he's his own worst enemy," or "she's her own worst enemy," or "I'm my own worst enemy" are very popular. It is very common and a sad commentary on how people learn to relate to themselves. Let's face it, they show themselves no mercy. And when someone gets sick

they can use that illness as another reason to feel bad about themselves.

In the previous experiment with the rats there was no scientific control animal. There were no rats hooked up with a dummy wire, a wire that carried no current. The following example includes genetically identical animals. Three rats are wired up as in the earlier example. Once again there is an empowered rat, one that can turn off the shock (Rat number 1). And also an unempowered rat (Rat number 2) who has to wait for his empowered relative to turn off the juice. Unlike the last experiment, one rat (Rat number 3) will have a mock wire. The wire is identical to the wire used to shock his brothers, but it is not hooked up to any current source. Therefore, no shock is administered to this rat. He is not experiencing the same shocking unfairness as the other two rats. Therefore, it seems that he would be the lucky one of the three rats.

Actually, not that lucky. In this experiment all three rats are given cancer. Their ability to reject the cancer will be tested. Recall that Rats 1 and 2 are getting shocked at random while Rat number 3 receives no shock whatsoever.

Logic would probably lead people to think that Rat number 3, the one not getting the bolus of electricity in his tail, would do the best job at rejecting the cancer. Here, logic fails in getting at the truth. It is Rat number 1 who has the least amount of cancer growth. Rat number 3, the one not getting shocked at all, is second in his ability to defend against the cancer. And Rat number 2, the unempowered rat, has the most cancer growth.

Isn't it interesting that Rat number 1 does better than Rat number 3? Rat number 1 is mobilizing some potential that allows his immune defense system to function better than the rat not getting shocked at all.

The Purpose and the Meaning

What is the purpose and meaning in the unfairness of life? Perhaps it has something to do with people accessing and expressing dormant abilities within themselves that would not be otherwise expressed. What is the meaning in the unfairness of a chronic illness? It is different for each individual patient. But holding the perspective that there is meaning allows them to have hope in spite of the prognosis.

Be hopeful that healing is possible. Offer that not to instill the false hope that a cure is coming, but instead offer that because it's the truth. Healing is possible because meaning offers people the perspective that includes the big picture. Life is a terminal condition. People all are destined for the same ultimate fate. And life is not fair. Hence, all people will be wounded by living as they experience the unfairness in a personal way. Wounds need to heal. Meaning often provides healing of their life wounds. Therefore, there is always hope.

And that healing can be and often is, inclusive of relationships within the family. When people are forced to confront the bigger issues of living, it provides everyone a broader view of reality. Human foibles are seen not so much as an indication of people's differences but instead, represent a reminder of their similarities. People no longer use the other person's idiosyncrasies as a distraction from doing what they can to serve and comfort. When clinicians open to their patients, in that warmth they have renewed hope.

Clinicians can become too focused on the disease and when a cure is not possible, lose hope. When clinicians lose hope, their patients can sense that and lose hope also. When a cure is not possible, they must remember their task as healers is not just to defeat the disease. It is to provide the best quality of life possible for their chronically ill patients.

Ways in which you might use the concept of hope in your practice and in turn instill hope in your chronically ill patients:

- Schedule an initial appointment of 90 minutes. Know that what your patients say has value and will be important in finding the meaning of the illness.

- Ask your patients what they think is the meaning of their illness. Ask them what physical, mental, and spiritual changes they wish to make, if any.
- This may be a beginning of a journey with your chronically ill patient. Allow time for them to get to know you. Invite them to participate in seminars or support groups that you are familiar with.
- You don't have control of who walks in your office. You will encounter patients who aren't pleasant. Do not take it personally. Instead, focus on responding to their needs in a way that truly serves the patient.

REFERENCES

1. *Alcoholics Anonymous*, p. 449.
2. Martin E.P. Seligman, *Learned Optimism*, Pocket Books, 1998, pp 168–170.

Chapter Six

Principle 3: Faith

John A. Mac Dougall

Now faith is the assurance of things hoped for, the conviction of things not seen.

Hebrews 11:1

Step Three and the Faith Principle

Step Three states: "Made a decision to turn our will and our lives over to the care of God as we understood Him."

■ THE ULTIMATE IMPORTANCE OF FAITH

An honest assessment of a chronic illness could lead to a lack of faith in medicine, faith in a Higher Power, and faith in the future, especially if people limit their ideas about possible outcomes to cure and failure. That is precisely why faith is necessary. The patient needs faith in their caregivers, family, and friends. They also need faith in a Higher Power and a process of recovery or healing although they may never be cured of their illness. They need faith that life can be fulfilling, even while chronically ill. Clinicians need faith in themselves, their skills, and colleagues and the system within which they work. They also need faith that a Higher Power is guiding the process. Faith is needed by both the clinician and the patient in order to trust the process. Their

Higher Power represents their faith. This Higher Power could be God, the natural healing process, or any other concept that provides hope.

■ THE CHALLENGE OF CHRONIC ILLNESS

Faith includes taking the challenge of chronic illness as an opportunity to examine not just physical health, but mental, emotional, and spiritual health as well. Having examined themselves with the clinician's help, patients need faith that something useful can be done to renew their lives. Faith is, by definition, about something that hasn't happened yet. They don't need faith about last Christmas because it is over. They only need faith that future Christmases will be good. To move from anxiety about a future state of well-being to a reality of help in the present, faith is needed that something will work.

The Benefits of Seeking a Higher Power

Faith is closely allied with hope. People begin to have faith that their hope will come true for them. Recovery and spiritual growth are not imposed on people by a Higher Power who knows what they need. Instead, they have to seek out their own recovery and spiritual growth. The experience of Alcoholics Anonymous (A.A.) was that seeking God was crucial. Their experience of confronting human limitations around alcoholism was true for all chronic illnesses. In the chapter "How It Works" in the book *Alcoholics Anonymous* they write,

> "a) That we were alcoholic and could not manage our own lives.
> b) That probably no human power could have relieved our alcoholism.
> c) That God could and would if He were sought."[1]

Faith is the belief that seeking a Higher Power is worthwhile and achievable. It is the willingness to have a relationship with a Higher Power that is important. People do not need great faith, or complete faith, just enough to get them moving. Whenever a friend or advisor suggests that they try something new, there is an element of faith in their positive response. The patient does not need to be sure the suggestion is right. They just need enough faith to try it.

Certainty versus Faith

Some people get stuck here. They seek certainty instead of simply having faith. In reality, certainty is rarely available. Most of decisions, routine and major, have to be taken with an element of faith. If they wait until 100 percent of the data is in, the time for a decision is probably long past. A common example is a decision to go to the movies. Often the decision is made with less than half of the information on what the movie is actually about. It's not possible to know everything about the movie in advance. For example, people can't be certain they will like the movie, but they can have faith that the movie will be good by reading the ads, the reviews, or intentionally selecting movies with a favorite actor, writer, or director. Although some movies are still disappointing, people continue to go to the movies because they have faith that it will be entertaining.

Prescribing Medication is No Easy Task

Every medication prescribed for patients has been determined to be likely to be safe and effective, but there is no advance proof that it will work. There is always the possibility that it will fail to work, or have side effects that outweigh the benefits.

■ **EDUCATED GUESSWORK**

Prescribing medication is guesswork. As my neurologist once said, "It's educated guesswork, but guesswork just the same."

After a hundred years of study, how aspirin works is only partially understood, but people take it all the time in the faith that it will help. For some uses, the feedback on aspirin comes quickly: pain is reduced or it isn't. For other uses, like prevention of heart attack, the feedback doesn't come at all. If there's no heart attack, that doesn't prove that aspirin prevented it. Many people find it wise to take it, even without proof or even clear evidence in one's own experience that it works. The group experience is taken, as reported in clinical trials, and decisions are based on that.

Women and Faith

There are some cultural reasons why faith comes more easily to women than to men. Because of the power imbalance that persists in society, women are better acquainted with the limits of their power, and the existence of powers greater than themselves. Men are more likely to see themselves as powerful, and thus less in need of a Higher Power. Religion and spirituality are seen as more a women's purview than a man's. Churches have a significant majority of women attending them. Women with children are often in charge of their children's spiritual development and religious instruction in a way that men aren't.

Is Spirituality Scientific?

There is a criticism from some patients at Hazelden that spirituality is unscientific. The benefits of healthy spirituality are firmly supported by the scientific method. For something to be scientific a theory is used. An experiment has been designed to demonstrate it. The experiment is conducted, the results counted, and then published. If the experiment can be duplicated, it is considered valid. A.A. experimented with different ways of obtaining a spiritual awakening as a treatment for alcoholism. They recorded their results as Twelve Steps and published them, in a book that describes the process and shares representative stories. Over the last sixty years, millions of men and women have successfully treated their alcoholism using these steps. They obtained much more than abstinence, they got a new way of life which is infinitely more satisfying than the old. Readers of these spiritual principles are invited to test them as guides for their behavior, and evaluate the results. It is a way for chronically ill patients to get in touch with spirituality, something they might not be familiar with.

Discovering Faith

Having obtained some hope for the future by seeing other people doing well, people find some faith that what worked for others may well work for them. They decide that they want what others have, and they begin to do what others did. People in Twelve Step programs call this taking the Third Step, which is "We made a decision to turn our will and our lives over to the care of God, *as we understood him.*"

This faith seems like a tall order, but it only calls for a decision that this is what they want to do. Turning their will and lives over seems like a total commitment that is beyond their grasp at that point. Such a commitment is scary, and summons up images of joining a mindless cult. However, they don't have to make a total commitment, simply a decision to enter into a different way of life. If they don't like the results, they can always stop.

It may help to realize that the words "our will" means thoughts, and the words "our lives" means actions. If they see life as a set of different relationships and issues, then on each issue and in each relationship, they practice turning their thoughts and actions over to the care of God, so that they can change.

In terms of a chronic illness, the words "our will" is what the person thinks about it and the words "our lives" is what they do about it. A person with a chronic illness might choose to take a helpful perspective that God cares for them and wishes to restore them. Chronic illness is not a failure of themselves or of God, but is part of the human condition. Bodies don't last forever, and they don't stay intact throughout their life. The illness is a part of them, a factor in their identity. Restoration may take the form of cure, comfort, or care, and healing comes in many forms. The Higher Power who created them can be their companion in the disease process.

A Shift in Thinking

If people believe that a chronic illness means that life isn't worthwhile, that comes true. A popular slogan holds true, "What I focus on, I become." If their thoughts are all about how the chronic illness defines them, and how life is bad, it becomes so. If they focus on being as well as they can be under the circumstances, they become better.

Many people with handicapping conditions have come to prefer the term "differently abled" to "disabled." This is because it represents a shift in how they think about themselves. If they are "disabled," the focus is on what they cannot do. If they are "differently abled" then the focus is on the fact that they are able to do things, but may need to do them differently. For a similar reason, hardly anyone uses the term "invalid" anymore. The noun "invalid" came to describe a person who had some difficulty carrying out normal activities, but the very term invalidated them as human beings.

■ THE BENEFITS OF UNDERSTANDING PAIN

I would prefer not to have chronic pain from migraine headaches, but there are some benefits. A major benefit is that it gives me an understanding of pain and the ability to hear it in others. It gives me compassion. It makes me a better counselor. I listen to the "red thread" of physical or emotional pain running through the other person's story, which gives me better insight. A minor benefit is that with a migraine it's easy to take my own pulse: I can hear it. The problems outweigh the benefits when I have the pain right in the moment. However, the benefits outweigh the problems when I don't have the pain right now.

Turning over my will means thinking of the headaches as simply part of who I am, rather than a sign of God's disfavor or abandonment. It also means accepting the reality that the migraines are often unpredictable, so there is no way of knowing whether the day will bring pain or not. I think of ways in which I can minimize the risk or impact of headaches, and of ways to live well anyhow.

Turning over my life means living in a way that is independent of the pain. This includes treating other people well, even when in pain. Just because I have a headache doesn't mean that everybody else has to have a figurative headache too. Turning over my life includes doing what I reasonably can to avoid or manage a headache, and then trusting God for the outcome.

Previously, I turned my will and my life over to the care of addictive drugs. I thought about maintaining my supply of sedatives and pain killers, about how to get a sympathetic doctor and a compliant pharmacy. The drugs didn't care for me well. Without killing the pain, I had blackouts and sometimes even passed out. Today, I take the new class of non-addictive migraine drugs, use relaxation techniques, massage, and biofeedback. I have been clean and sober for 10 years. This prevents "rebound" headaches from drug withdrawal. When in pain, I take the safe medication, lie down with a cloth blindfold to block out the light, and meditate, either to music or in a conversation with God. I have let go of anger with God for the lack of a cure, and opened up to care: self-care, the care of other people, and the care of God.

Turning It Over: A Form of Mobile Meditation

People turning their will and lives over to the care of God makes sense on a wide range of issues. Gradually, it becomes a form of mobile meditation. As each issue or theme arises throughout the day, they check out their thoughts and actions, and open them to the care of their Higher Power. For instance, if they tried this within marriage, they would ask God to guide what they think about their spouse and what they do with them. This would make it difficult to treat them badly. In turn, if they tried this at work, they would invite God to direct what they think about employers, co-workers, and customers. It would make God their ultimate employer. If people turned their will and lives over while driving, it would end road rage. Competition would be replaced with courtesy. If they applied this to their relationships with people who annoyed them, their resentments would be lessened.

The Danger of Resentment

A.A. recognized the risk of holding onto resentments against others. Although the targets of resentments may not be injured by feelings of resentment, the resentment makes the person with those feelings sicker. Their disease becomes more powerful as a result and they move towards relapse. In the chapter "Freedom From Bondage" A.A. quotes a clergyman's prescription: not just for resentments but for the prevention of the relapse that resentments cause:

> "If you have a resentment you want to be free of, if you will pray for that person or the thing that you resent, you will be free. Ask for their health, their prosperity, their happiness, and you will be free. Even when you don't really want it for them, and your prayers are only words and you don't mean it, go ahead and do it anyway. Do it every day for two weeks and you will find you have come to mean it and to want it for them,

and you will realize that where you used to feel bitterness and resentment and hatred, you now feel compassionate understanding and love."[2]

■ HIGHER POWER: THE SPIRITUAL CORE

Everyone has a spiritual core. This is the organizing principle at the heart of thoughts and actions. The spiritual core is related to the nature of the person's Higher Power. Who or what their Higher Power is influences their thoughts and actions. In turn, their choice of thoughts and actions influence their choice of a Higher Power. If their addiction is their Higher Power, their thoughts will be of drugs and their actions will be organized around maintaining a supply, both inside and outside of their bodies. If people don't know they are addicts, their behavior may not make sense. Once they know what their Higher Power is, the pieces fall into place and they become predictable. If money is their Higher Power, they will be greedy in attitude and behavior. Others will notice the influence of the "Almighty Dollar" in their lives, and begin to move away. They will be loyal to whatever makes them richer.

Power itself can be a person's Higher Power. Winning becomes their goal in all circumstances. In turn, they try to conquer others in their relationships instead of loving them. If their nationality or religion is their Higher Power, they are likely to have conflict with people who are unlike them, convinced that they are doing God's will. If they believe they are God's chosen, then they will determine that all others must be wrong. If they choose their own ego as their Higher Power, then their thoughts will be focused on themselves. Other people will have meaning only to the extent they bolster their ego. The egocentric person may state, "Well, that's enough about me. What about you? What do you think of me?"

Illnesses can become a person's Higher Power. If this occurs, illness will be used as their defining feature. The least healthy parts of themselves become who they are. Illness provides a self-definition, an excuse for anything they don't want to do, and a reproach against the rest of the world for the way life has not satisfied them. Sex can also be their chosen Higher Power. If so, it dominates their thoughts, feelings, and behaviors.

■ NEGATIVE AND POSITIVE HIGHER POWERS

There is a big difference between a negative and positive Higher Power. With any negative Higher Power, things are loved and people are used. With a positive Higher Power, people are loved and things are used. Religions or spiritual programs that are healthy result in all people being valued because they have a God of restoration and care. When people make a decision that they want this positive Higher Power for their own, their thoughts and actions, their will and lives, become loving towards God, themselves, and others. Their Higher Power is at the center of their lives. It also energizes them, and the spirit of their Higher Power becomes their own.

■ DECISIONS AND BEHAVIOR MODIFICATION

Making a decision doesn't make that decision come true. For example, two patients with coronary artery disease might make the same decision to carry out a heart healthy lifestyle. One might make the decision, but not follow it with any changed behavior. Thus the decision becomes as transient as most New Year's resolutions. The other might change his diet, carry out moderate exercise, stop smoking, and begin to live a life that is based on the spiritual principles outlined here, rather than a life dominated by struggle against time, people, places, and things. As he does these things, his decision comes true. The same holds true with spiritual growth. Having decided, people need to summon up their courage, and change their behaviors.

Having developed the faith to turn their will and lives over to the care of God, they need to know how to do it. Understanding their will as thoughts and their lives as actions, they resolve to invite their Higher Power to guide both. It is tempting to try a "one big decision" method, going for a sudden spiritual awakening as the result of one prayer. That might happen, but for most people they will have a gradual spiritual awakening as they grow. Patients should be encouraged to do the same.

Try to trust that things are working out the way they should, for you and for your patients.

Suggestions for faith in your life and work:

- Consider your own Higher Power(s). In whom or what do you have faith? Make a list. It might include God, yourself, your clinical skills, your colleagues, research, and the healing process.
- Make a decision to turn your will and your life over to the care of God, as you understand God.
- Ask your patients about their Higher Powers. In whom do they have faith? Is it God, you, their family, prayers, medicine, therapy, pets, friends, or something else?
- If your patients believe in God, ask about what they believe God's will is for them.

Bowen F. White

Faith is an important strand of the knot. It is a belief in something greater than oneself. An August 9, 1999 *U.S. News & World Report* article cites a Duke University study where 4,000 elderly people who attend weekly religious services are 28 percent less likely to die in a 7-year period. Through their faith, people know that regardless of all their failings, they are accepted as a member of the family of God. In that family there is no "if" clause. It's not, if they're somehow more perfect people, then they will be more worthy of family of God membership.

People are not used to that kind of relationship with anything but the family dog. Even with their own children there may be an "if" clause. There are bumper stickers in many communities that read: "Proud Parent of Honor Roll Student at Maplewood School." The "if" clause in this statement implies if the child makes good grades then the adult will be proud to be their parent. If they clean their room, if they score the goal, if they get the part, if they win the prize, if they become an eagle scout, then parents will be proud of their children.

■ IMPLICATIONS OF THE "IF" CLAUSE

You know, I don't want there to be an "if" clause in my relationships with my children. If there is an "if" clause in my relationships with my four daughters, then they will probably only share their victories and successes with me.

But, when things are going well, how much do they really need my support? My belief is that when they really need my support is when things are going poorly. I want them to know that they can count on me to be there for them regardless of what they have done. More than that, I want them to know that they are treasures in my eyes. They are treasures regardless of what they do or don't do. Regardless of what mistakes they have made, I thank heaven every day that I am their father. This is what I want my relationship with my children to be.

And I want my relationships with my chronically ill patients to be similar. I want them to have faith in me and know that I am not going to leave "if" they neglect to take their medication or follow their exercise plan. I am there for the good times and the bad. I am making a commitment to the patient regardless of how the illness progresses. I want my patient to feel comfortable with me and be open about how they are feeling not only physically, but emotionally, and spiritually. This is one of the reasons why I feel it is important to know about my patient's belief system. I ask the patient if they believe in God. If they don't, I ask them what they believe in. Sometimes they don't know. If they don't have an answer, I further prompt them by asking them if they believe in love. If they answer yes, I point out that they have experienced something they can't prove the existence of.

I believe that pure religion is love in action. I then ask the patient what they might want to change in their lives in terms of their love relationships. That includes their relationship with themselves. This gets them to open up. If I go on talking about God and they don't believe in God, then I am shutting the door on my patient instead of opening it. When talking about faith, it is important to approach the topic with an open mind and not pre-judge the patient for their belief system.

If you do not believe in God, that is fine. You will still want to broach the subject of your patient's faith. It will help you understand where they are coming from and the reasoning behind some of their decisions. Whatever their faith, it is important to be respectful of their belief system.[3]

Faith is important to me not only as a physician, but as a human being. Often, I lose faith in myself. Therefore, I need support to get back up after I fall. I need something greater than myself to help me reconnect. I need to have faith that I can be vulnerable, reveal myself, and ask for what I need and expect to receive it. I expect mercy. Luke 11:9 states, "Ask and it shall be given to you." Mercy—it heals.

Merciless

Often, people are merciless with themselves. They are self critical, judgmental, and demeaning to themselves. It is amazing how their own secret thoughts can overwhelm them. The Bible talks about asking for mercy and receiving it. Humans are built to be imperfect beings. If people make mistakes, they won't be denied mercy, no matter what they've done. There is no "if" clause for mercy. There is an incredible sense of comfort once people recognize this.

■ AN EYE-OPENING EXPERIENCE

I once heard author Joseph Campbell talk about his book, *A Skeleton Key To Finnegan's Wake*.[4] In this book he interpreted the symbolism of James Joyce's animal allegory *Finnegan's Wake*.[5] In the Joyce book, the numbers 11 and 32 keep coming up over and over. Joseph interpreted the symbology of these numbers in his book. About 5 years later he had an eye-opening experience while teaching a group of students a class on the New Testament.

He was preparing for the class, reading Paul's letters to the Romans. He came upon this passage, "Lord you have created us to be disobedient so that you could show us your mercy." And he looked over and saw it was Romans 11:32. Ah ha, 11:32, it was then that he realized his former interpretation was mistaken. This is what Joyce was referring to in his work. And Campbell did not discover it until that moment.

What this passage says to me, is what it said to Campbell and probably what it said to Joyce. Mercy cannot be denied us because God created us to be disobedient. God set up the arrangement to allow humans to screw up, which we do. We get in trouble and need help. And God has to help us when we ask because we are set up to mess everything up. The ultimate help that we are offered is mercy. And it is ours for the asking. But we have to ask.

There is no "if" clause. If you pray five times a day, then you get mercy. If you go to church twice a week, then you get mercy. It is, regardless of what heinous deeds you have done, mercy is yours for the asking. It is our divine inheritance, our birthright in the family of God.

Now, how often can we rely on this safety net? That depends upon your faith. My belief is that forgiveness and mercy can never be withheld from us. We were made to be disobedient. It's in our bones. Hence, when we ask for forgiveness we have to be forgiven.

In Matthew 18:22 Peter asks Jesus how many times should someone be forgiven. Jesus says 70 times seven. That's advice for us clay-footed folks. If we are to forgive people four hundred and ninety times, how often should the Supreme Being forgive us? An infinite number, no limit, that is my belief. Amazing Grace indeed. Mercy, Mercy, Mercy.

Dealing with the Chronically Ill Patient

Some things a clinician should consider when dealing with a chronically ill patient include: Can they talk to their patients about their faith? Can they ask them to share with them how they are using their faith as a resource for healing their lives? Is prayer an important part of their faith? Are they willing to share with their patients the data that shows how prayer can be healing? Larry Dossey, M.D., researched the literature and found many scientific studies to verify the value of prayer in healing. His books *Reinventing Medicine* and *Healing Words*[6] are good resources for clinicians. If asked, would the clinicians share their faith with the suffering people that they see? If their answer is "no" and they are unwilling to share their faith in an open, non-judgmental way, patients may not be able to open up and let them see that part of the knot for them. If their answer is yes, but they attempt to force their faith on patients in a rigid, judgmental way, then what they are doing is demeaning. It is disrespectful and the opposite of healing. And, isn't healing what they came to see the clinician for?

■ DELIGHTFUL GERTIE

When I was growing up, there was a wonderful woman that came into our household to help my mom with the housework and child-care duties. Her name was Gertie. She was born in 1896 and first worked for my folks in the 1940s. She never had any children of her own. We were her children. She loved us and we loved her. I think she was a saint. She was always pleasant, had an easy smile that quickly broke into a delightful laugh. And it was easy to make her laugh.

After I grew up, got married, went to medical school, had children, finished a family practice residency, hung up my shingle, built a practice, many years had gone by. Gertie got older too. She kept working for my folks until she was over ninety years old. Then she went into a nursing home. I went to visit her there.

I took a bag with some fun stuff in it to play with Gertie and her friends. Gertie was in a room with five or six beds. I looked in from the doorway and could see someone sitting in a wheelchair by a big window. No one else was in the room. At first, I wasn't sure it was Gertie as she was sitting with her back to the door. Standing there, I saw a small woman sitting caddywhompous in a wheelchair. Her black wig was also sideways on her head and matted white hair was exposed on one side. She was kneading the window curtain with her hands and rocking back and forth. The smell of urine was prevalent in the stale air. I walked up slowly as I didn't want to startle her and I wanted to make sure it was Gertie.

As I approached, I could hear that she was speaking as she rocked. It was Gertie. As I arrived by her side, I couldn't quite hear what she was saying. But, the whole thing was very depressing. I was thinking about how sad it was to see this woman in this way. She had been so important to me and had taught me so much.

I bent closer to hear what she was saying as she rocked, eyes closed, kneading the curtain. Her voice was soft, just above a whisper, but clear. She was repeatedly saying, "Thank you Jesus, Mercy, Mercy, Jesus, thank you, thank you." Over and over, this was her mantra. She did not notice my tears when she looked up, glasses off one ear, at me.

"Who is that?" she inquired.

"It's me, Bowen." I replied.

"Bowen, is that you child?" she asked loudly.

"Yes, Gertie, it's me. I've come to visit and play with you and your friends," I answered. "Come down here where I can get a good look at you," she said with authority.

I straightened her heavy, coke bottle glasses and kneeled next to her chair. We talked a while. Her cognition was intact, then it would lapse. She went in and out. I straightened her wig and helped get her properly placed in the chair. Then I wheeled her out to the great room. We put all the wheelchairs in a circle and got everyone involved in some sort of silliness. We had a great time.

The staff was grateful. They could see how much fun we were having and encouraged me to return. I left having had a fabulous time with my old friend and teacher. I planned to come back. But, I never did. I got distracted and Gertie died not long thereafter.

Driving off I thought, how perfect. Gertie was fading, body and mind failing, yet there she was teaching me once again. It was depressing for me to see her there rocking by the window. But, she wasn't depressed. She was ecstatic. She was showing me by example a faith that was constant, that allowed her to keep some sense of balance at the end of her life. She was focused on the knot and it was pulling her toward it. Her spirit was a shining example for me. "Mercy, Mercy, Mercy!"

Ways in which you can incorporate faith in your life and address the topic of faith with your patients:

- Ask your patient about their religious/spiritual beliefs and listen to what they have to say. If they claim to not have religious beliefs, approach the topic differently.
- Don't push your religious/spiritual beliefs onto the patient. Respect their beliefs.
- Pray with your patient if they request you to do so and you are comfortable with it.
- Use your own faith to guide you as you treat the infirm. Pray for guidance before you greet your patient.

NOTES AND REFERENCES

1. *Alcoholics Anonymous*, p. 449.
2. Ibid., p. 552.

3. The National Institute for Healthcare Research (NIHR) conducts and coordinates research on the relationship between spirituality and physical and mental health. The president, David Larson, M.D. believes physicians are ready to accept spirituality into their treatment plans if good science backs it up.
4. Joseph Campbell, *A Skeleton Key to Finnegan's Wake*, Harcourt Brace, New York, 1944.
5. James Joyce, *Finnegan's Wake*, Viking Press, New York, 1939.
6. Larry Dossey, *Healing Words: The Power of Prayer and the Practice of Medicine*, Harper, San Francisco, 1995.

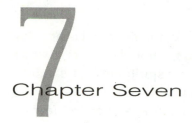

Chapter Seven

Principle 4: Courage

John A. Mac Dougall

> The life which is unexamined is not worth living.
> Plato, *Dialogues*, section 38

Step Four and the Courage Principle

Step Four states: "Made a searching and fearless moral inventory of ourselves."

▪ A COURAGEOUS SELF-EXAMINATION

Most religions have some form of spiritual self-examination. By examining conscience, the fact that conscience exists is brought forth. Because this is often an unpleasant examination people often avoid doing it. To claim spiritual progress, they take an honest look at themselves, with hope that it will lead to change, and faith that their Higher Power is ready to help them correct what they find. A courageous self-examination is in order.

The Fourth Step of Twelve Step programs reads: "They took a searching and fearless moral inventory of themselves." This is a "we" step. It is something that everyone who lives an examined life does, not once, but periodically over a lifetime. Taking this step gets people out of isolation and into a process of personal growth. This conscience examination is appropriate for the physician or other clinician, as well as for the patient. One of the risks of being a professional caregiver is the development of the belief that clinicians are very different from their patients. An examination of how medical professionals conduct their clinical practices, according to these spiritual principles, should happen before proposing to help their patients with their spirituality, and should continue on an ongoing basis. They cannot give what they do not have. Both doctor and patient need the courage to examine their own lives.

■ A SEARCHING AND MORAL INVENTORY

A searching examination of conscience should take place. For chronic illness patients of any kind, it should include a careful examination into the ways they may have contributed to the illness, neglected to care for themselves well over its course, and any thought or behavior patterns that block recovery. Sometimes they have played no role at all in their illness. At other times they have. A searching and fearless inventory is needed to find out.

In addition to an inventory of how they participated in the origins or continuation of their chronic illness, they need to inventory their thoughts and behaviors towards other people, themselves, and their Higher Power. What are they thinking and doing that truly enhances their relationships with God, self, and others? What is it about their will and their lives that split those apart?

A "fearless" moral inventory can be difficult. For many people, this can be interpreted as a reason to postpone this process, or avoid it altogether. If they still have fear, they rationalize that they must not be fearless, and so they aren't ready. However, the longer they put it off the more fearful they are likely to become, and so it becomes ever harder to become "fearless."

■ REDEFINING FEARLESS

I finally got past this point in my process by redefining fearless. Instead of "no fear at all," I define "fearless" for the purposes of this step as acknowledging my fear, setting it aside, and going on. Courage is not the absence of fear. It is doing the right thing, even when afraid. What is the right thing?

■ THE NATURE OF RIGHT AND WRONG

The examination of conscience should be a moral inventory. Most people take part in a broad consensus on the nature of right and wrong. In addition, whatever leads them towards the best possible health is right for them, and whatever leads them towards a chronic illness relapse is wrong for them. For example, having two beers while someone mows the lawn is not immoral, unless they're an alcoholic. Then it is morally wrong because it precipitates a relapse in their alcoholism. Having a filet mignon, baked potato and sour cream, followed by a hot fudge ice cream sundae isn't morally wrong, but if the person has coronary artery disease it may be wrong for them because it makes the damage worse.

Some typical gender differences must be considered in an examination of conscience. For men, wrongdoing often consists of violating rules, laws, or societal expectations. Wrongdoing is likely to consist of something they did that injures other people. For women, wrongdoing often consists of not taking action to live up to their full potential. Believing themselves incapable, or deferring to others, keeps them from being all they could be. For women, doing wrong often is more subtle, consisting of not doing something that would have benefited them or others.

With a chronic illness, the first question on the patient's moral inventory is "Have we had a searching and fearless physical inventory?" Many of them who are ill have not had a real physical exam by a physician who might know about their condition.

■ "I'D RATHER NOT KNOW"

One woman told me about some of her symptoms which were all symptoms of multiple sclerosis. At her last physical examination, the physician suggested she slow down and get plenty of rest. When I inquired further, she confessed, "He wanted me to take the test for multiple sclerosis, but there's not much they can do about it, so I told him I'd rather not know."

■ THE HARMFULNESS OF NOT KNOWING

In many cases, what people don't know can hurt them. Many people avoid seeking any kind of physical exam, lest they find out something is wrong. Having no information means that their denial of aging and illness is undisturbed. Or, having been diagnosed and treated for a chronic illness such as high blood pressure, they simply go off the medicine on the grounds that they don't feel bad, and never check again. Smokers often avoid any doctor because they fear the confrontation that is likely to come over their smoking.

■ INDIFFERENCE

In some cases, even people who have been confronted with misconduct never think to look for a physical cause. I had a ministerial colleague who was on the verge of being dismissed. He was charged with "indifference to the work of the ministry." He slept a lot and was sluggish when awake, doing little work in his parish. I convinced his wife to get him to a doctor for a physical (an earlier attempt to deal directly with the minister had failed). He was found to be diabetic. His blood sugar so high he was almost comatose. Neither he nor his church had thought of a physical inventory.

Having identified both illnesses and risk factors of it, we then need to inventory those of our behaviors that keep us sick or make us worse. I had, for many years, done exactly the wrong thing for migraines. I treated them with alcohol and other drugs and didn't mobilize to face my problems. Some forms of alcohol directly made the headaches worse, such as red wine. All the drugs I took, including the alcohol, were depressants: tranquilizers and narcotics. As a result, I avoided taking action on issues that were painful. I was left with painful thoughts and feelings that were unresolved.

One cause of my migraines was drug withdrawal and rebound headaches. Another was the transformation of painful thoughts and feelings into physical pain. Both tended to hit their peak around 11 a.m. The result was that I had a migraine every day, from at least 11 a.m. on, for seven years. Nothing changed until the doctor who was so generous with those addictive drugs died, and the new doctor asked, "Are you taking all this medicine?" (Yes.) "Do you still have a headache?'' (Yes.) ''Do you know what that means?'' (No.) ''It means the medicine isn't working.'' (Oh) Of course, by then I was an addict, and simply cut down on the brands of drugs I was taking, and settled on two. I found another doctor for those prescriptions. Even when I quit drinking and drugging, it was to treat addiction, not migraines. Only after I had been sober for four years did I inquire into a thorough assessment at a headache clinic.

The oddest thing about my headache recovery is that, for months after being supplied with a safe and effective drug for direct treatment, I failed to carry it with me. The fact that it was an injection and meant carrying a kit provided an excuse. However, whenever the pain struck, I would curse myself for forgetting it. The cursing probably didn't help. Now I am well supplied, and keep what I need on hand. I have medication, a cloth blindfold for light, and music for relaxation at home, in my office, and in a briefcase or computer case when I travel. Finally, I am cooperating in my own recovery. Our behaviors and the spiritual states that drive them can make us healthier or sicker. Many physical illnesses can be created with disturbances in behavior or relationships. Illnesses, although entirely real, can also be metaphors for our spiritual state.

■ LETTING GO OF ANGER

One man in chemical dependency treatment was doing adequately in identifying his alcoholism and taking responsibility for his sobriety. However, his counselor was struck by the level of anger at the world and at certain targets: gays, police officers, newspaper editors, and ex-wives. The man completed his assignments in treatment, but the counselor told him: ''You've got to do something about letting go of your anger, or you head's going to blow up.'' Six months later the patient was dead of a cerebral hemorrhage. He was sober, but his head blew up.

■ THE IMPORTANCE OF SELF-CARE

I counseled a woman who was a middle-aged, traditional, Italian-American homemaker. She was the ''shock absorber'' in her extended family. She listened to all sides in their feuds, cushioned the children from the rages of their father, did everything possible to ensure the family's happiness, and managed the family rituals. By the time her children were grown, she was still performing all these functions for her adult children. She was tired, and developed a case of fibromyalgia in her shoulders that ended up with her in the hospital. In talking with her, I observed that she had been carrying the weight of the world on her shoulders for years, so no wonder they hurt. She took a variety of actions: medication, rest, and physical therapy. She also began to shed some of her responsibilities. The family was horrified the first time she refused to cook and clean up a lavish Thanksgiving dinner for everyone (she did offer to bake the turkey). They adjusted and the combination of different forms of care and self-care alleviated her disease. It has not gone entirely away, but it is much better.

■ BUILDING A PROTECTIVE SHELL

Some survivors of physical or sexual abuse distort their body shapes without being fully aware of what they are doing or the consequences. By starving until they are exceptionally thin, survivors can eliminate their sexual desirability and become literally less of a target. By adding weight until they are dreadfully obese, others guarantee a lack of sexual attractiveness and also add padding that feels a lot like protection. Alan D., whose spiritual issues were fear and abandonment as a result of child abuse, persistently failed in his efforts to lose weight. Whenever he did lose weight, he would become both anxious and hungry. He finally figured out that the forty extra pounds he carried felt like protection against abuse. He even joked that, "If somebody tries to hurt me, I can always fall on them." He once worked as a cab driver and wore a bulletproof vest in the city. His extra weight felt kind of like that to him. Once he did an inventory of his behaviors around weight, he started doing massage therapy with a woman who specialized in abuse survivors. Within five months he had lost eighteen pounds, and was not having anxiety about the prospect of losing more.

■ LOOKING BEYOND THE DRUGS OR THE ILLNESS

Alcoholics and addicts who only try to treat their drinking and drugging without addressing the patterns of beliefs and behaviors that drive them, are likely to relapse again and again. The Twelve Step programs are not programs about "not drinking." That's the milk carton program, "Just say no." It works for a while, and then the addict or alcoholic just says yes, and the problem recurs. Narcotics Anonymous' big contribution to the field of recovery is the realization that it's not the drug that's the problem. The problem is "between your ears." That is, the physical, mental, emotional, and spiritual state of being an addict is the problem, not the drugs.

As people inventory their chronic illness, it is good to note the physical, mental, emotional, and spiritual aspects of the disease. As they inventory themselves as part of recovery, all these factors need to be included. They need to know the whole truth about their lives.

■ EXAMINING CONSCIENCE THROUGH WRITING

The examination of conscience is best done in writing. Writing provokes thinking. Many ideas and insights will come while writing that would never arise by just sitting and thinking. People may choose privacy while they write. The results of this examination are to be shared only with their Higher Power and one other human being. It is not to be immediately shared with everybody. Later they can choose to share what's appropriate with others.

■ A QUEST FOR SPIRITUAL GROWTH

There are many suggested ways of spiritual self-examination, such as the spiritual exercises of St. Ignatius Loyola or a number of Fourth Step guides. However, a few key topics can get people started in their quest for spiritual growth.

■ THE TROUBLE WITH RESENTMENTS

Resentments are always trouble because they are a powerful form of attachment. Through resentments people are bound to institutions or people that harm them. If people have a good reason for their resentments, the situation is even worse because they're likely to keep the resentments because they're "right." Even if they're right about the situation, they're wrong to keep the resentment because it injures them. At a minimum, they're giving a lot of time and attention to someone or something that's a burden on their lives. A healthier response is to detach from people, places, and things that are bad for them, and attach to those who are good for them.

Alcoholics Anonymous (A.A.) gives their reasons why resentments are a block to happiness and even to survival:

> "It is plain that a life which includes deep resentment leads only to futility and unhappiness. To the precise extent that we permit these, do we squander the hours that might have been worth while. But with the alcoholic, whose hope is in the maintenance and growth of a spiritual experience, this business of resentment is infinitely grave.
>
> We found that it is fatal. For when harboring such feelings we shut ourselves off from the sunlight of the Spirit. The insanity of alcohol returns and we drink again. And with us, to drink is to die."[1]

When people focus on their resentments, they are "letting others live rent free in their head." The voices of the accumulated resentments are sometimes called "the committee of idiots." It is best not to listen to them. One slogan for getting rid of resentments is, "I've got to stop auctioning myself off to the low bidder." By thinking about people who are bad for them, they are "auctioning themselves off" to them because they dominate their thoughts and feelings. Alan D. reached a sticking point in his recovery. His justifiable anger over being abused as a child had curdled into major resentments against his abusers, some of whom were still alive. In A.A., he read the chapter "Freedom from Bondage" about praying for them. He couldn't do it. He did, however, pray about the resentments. He perceived the voice of his Higher Power saying to him: "You can get well or you can get even. Pick one." He picked getting well, and the resentments began to fade. It took years, but they are now over.

■ ASKING THE RIGHT QUESTIONS

Whom do we resent? Why? Did we play any part in creating the problem that is the basis of our resentments? What institutions or events do we resent? What power are we giving them? How have our resentments affected us? A spiritual self-examination isn't all negative. When a store takes inventory, they count what remains, not just what's gone. We need to consider the positives in our inventory. The opposite of resentment is tolerance, patience, and open-mindedness. These improve our relationships with Higher Power, self, and others. They can be a treatment for resentment, especially if combined with prayer and meditation. So how have we practiced tolerance, patience, and open-mindedness? With whom? What were the results?

■ THE STRESS AND ISOLATION OF DISHONESTY

Dishonesty contributes to chronic illness. At a minimum, a pattern of dishonesty creates stress and isolation. A result of conflict with people is that they go away. Stress plays a part in many illnesses and creates fatigue. Isolation may seem desirable, especially when the person is filled with resentment and conflict. However, people aren't made to live in isolation. One of the worst punishments society inflicts is solitary confinement.

A.A. makes this statement about the importance of honesty for spiritual growth:

> "Those who do not recover are people who cannot or will not completely give themselves to this simple program, usually men and women who are constitutionally incapable of being honest with themselves."[2]

Only those who are spiritually well can prosper alone. When they're dishonest, they're not spiritually well. If they are habitually dishonest, they'll be dishonest about their chronic illness as well, and be cut off from help.

A basic form of dishonesty is self-deception. After people have successfully lied to themselves, they begin to believe their own stories. In turn, lying to others is easy. Their compass is altered. Instead of the needle pointing to the true north of reality, it points now to whatever is the most convenient. Sometimes loving but ill-informed family members will lie to a seriously sick person because they "do not want to upset them." This dishonesty isolates the sick person at a time when they need fellowship the most and gets in the way of effective care planning.

■ QUESTIONS TO ASK ABOUT DISHONESTY

How have we been dishonest, both with ourselves and with others? What stories do we tell that aren't true? With whom have we been dishonest? What are the effects of our dishonesty on our self-esteem, ambitions, personal, and sexual relationships?

■ HONESTY: AN ATTITUDE OF TRUTH, FAIRNESS, AND HELPFULNESS TOWARDS OTHERS

For a balanced inventory, people also consider the ways in which they have been honest, and assess the results. How have they been honest, and what have been the effects of their honesty, on themselves and on others? Not all honesty heals. Sometimes aggression is disguised as honesty, sometimes called being "brutally honest." So while assessing their honesty, it is important to make sure that the desire is to live in harmony with others, not to use it as a weapon.

Honesty is more than being factually accurate. It can be inaccurate and still be honest, as in "an honest mistake." Honesty is an attitude of truth, fairness, and helpfulness towards others. It includes being truthful and consistent while refraining from taking unfair advantage of others. With an honest person, what you see is what you get.

Fear is usually harmful. Some fear is legitimate, and protects people from danger. Fear of falling is useful for someone on the edge of a cliff, but it is a burden if their employment requires a lot of flying, standing on a ladder or perching in high places cleaning windows. Fear can also be taken beyond its intended purpose as a safety device and made into a Higher Power, or a governing part of people's lives where it has no useful purpose.

■ FEAR ISN'T A GOOD BASIS FOR CAREFUL PLANNING

An unfortunate business management style is called "Management by Crisis." It goes like this: the business has a crisis and the management reacts out of fear of harm, and institutes policies to manage it. The solution to the crisis becomes the origin of the next crisis because fear isn't a good basis for careful planning. A case in point: Shortly before one large company went bankrupt, it fired most of the secretaries to save money. While the short-term financial crisis was resolved, during the following 90 days, the engineers lacked support and couldn't find anything. As a result, their work wasn't completed in time. The solution to this crisis became the origin of the next crisis. This also happens on an individual level when people lie their way out of a problem. The lies they've told to avoid the problem usually become the source of the next problem.

A.A. speaks of fear as a persistent theme in life, both a problem and a cause of new problems:

> "This short word somehow touches about every aspect of our lives. It was an evil and corroding thread; the fabric of our existence was shot through with it. It set in motion trains of circumstances, which brought us misfortune we felt we didn't deserve. But did not we, ourselves, set the ball rolling? Sometimes we think fear ought to be classed with stealing. It seems to cause more trouble."[3]

■ THE PHYSIOLOGICAL ASPECTS OF FEAR

What fear does to people's physiology is obvious: perspiration, rapid breathing, upset stomach, and many other symptoms can come from fear. What is less obvious is what does not happen: when they are afraid, they disengage from life. They don't stretch and try new activities or relationships. They don't take risks. With a lack of risk comes a lack of reward, and life becomes less rewarding. What are they afraid of? How reasonable are their fears? How likely are they to come true? What opportunities have they passed up because of their fears? What important things have they left unsaid because they fear the disapproval of others? What are the effects of their fears on them, their hopes, and their relationships?

■ THE POSITIVE CHOICE: TRUST

Trust is the more positive choice in the face of fear. People need to learn to build trust with trustworthy people, with themselves, and with a Higher Power. They build trust through carefully chosen risks and the evaluation of the relationships within which they take the risks. To build durable trust with other people, they first share something that is a little bit intimate with them. If the others listen thoughtfully, without interruption, gossip, or rejection, they can conclude that the others are likely to be trustworthy. If they then begin to share some of their own feelings, it becomes a good sign because true trust is a two way street. People then risk a little more and reevaluate the situation. People build trust with others based on their experiences with them. Trust is built in themselves by trying out new behaviors and then evaluating the results. When people risk, they may gain not only the thing they risked to get, but also an increased sense of trust in themselves. They can be mistaken without being wrong. As long as they are loyal to themselves, they can tolerate honest mistakes without shaking their basic trust.

Similarly, people build trust in their Higher Power through prayer and meditation. They place themselves in contact with their Higher Power and entrust themselves to God's care. They then evaluate how life is going. If they experience themselves as being cared for, then they trust more.

A.A. speaks of the value of trust in a Higher Power:

> "We never apologize to anyone for depending upon our Creator. We can laugh at those who think spirituality the way

of weakness. Paradoxically, it is the way of strength. The verdict of the ages is that faith means courage."[4]

■ **QUESTIONS ABOUT TRUST**

How have we demonstrated trust in ourselves, friends and family, a Twelve Step Program, our health care providers, and a Higher Power? Whom do we trust? Can we trust that we are consistently looking out for our own best interest, or do we still have elements of self-sabotage?

■ **MIXED MESSAGES**

How people express their sexuality is worthy of careful self-examination. American society has an interesting contrast. While there are great volumes of sexually oriented material on television and in the movies, little of it is useful for guidance. Many television shows rely on tasteless jokes that the viewers would be ashamed to tell, but they are willing to watch nonetheless. Viewers receive lots of information on sexuality but very little wisdom about it.

A.A. has a useful standard for taking an inventory of our sexual relationships:

> "We reviewed our own conduct over the years past. Where had we been selfish, dishonest, or inconsiderate? Whom had we hurt? Did we unjustifiably arouse jealousy, suspicion, or bitterness? Where were we at fault, and what should we have done instead? They got this all down on paper and looked at it. In this way we tried to shape a sane and sound ideal for our future sex life. We subjected each relation to this test—was it selfish or not?"[5]

Examining Sexual Relationships

How have people been selfish in their sexual relationships? How have they used other people, instead of loving them? They can usually find rationalizations why their behavior wasn't so bad, but an inventory isn't about explaining away their behavior, it's about carefully examining it. One guide to whether a relationship is exploitive is to explore the relationship between the level of sexual intimacy and the level of commitment. If the level of sexual intimacy exceeds the level of commitment, then they are probably using the other person. Very few people today still believe in the idea of sex as harmless fun. When people have sex with someone without much of a commitment, it is unlikely to stay harmless.

How have people allowed themselves to be used by others? Sometimes there is a pattern of mutual exploitation in sexual relationships, instead of love and care. Before feminism, young women were routinely taught to trade their sexuality for economic security instead of seeking the means to become economically secure themselves. Some people exchange sex for drugs. Nobody's really in love in this situation as both parties have ulterior motives. Sometimes people have sex with someone they don't really love just because they want the attention and don't want to be alone. While one person is taking care of their sexual desire, the other person is dealing with their loneliness. This is not an example of a relationship of mutual commitment and care.

It might be worth examining how people have they been unselfish in their sexual relations. Used correctly, sexuality is a gift of love, tenderness, pleasure, and comfort. If they're lucky, two people can give and receive at the same time. Sometimes timing is off and the giving is more one way. But, as long as commitment and trust characterize the overall relationship, then the relationship is unselfish.

Family Relationships and Chronic Illness

Family relationships are important. Any chronic illness is a burden on the family if only because of the practical considerations of arranging for caregiving and taking care of special needs. Unfortunately, the chronically ill sometimes make their family's burden even worse by their own unkind behavior when they are feeling ill. This is more obvious with the alcoholic or addict, but people who have many other chronic illnesses take out the stress of the situation on their families. While some with emotional, mental, or neurological illness can't help it, others can, but continue inflicting their own pain on their families.

A.A. acknowledges the damage the alcoholic can cause:

> "The alcoholic is like a tornado roaring his way through the lives of others. Hearts are broken. Sweet relationships are dead. Affections have been uprooted. Selfish and inconsiderate habits have kept the home in turmoil."[6]

■ **QUESTIONS TO ASK**

How have we injured family and friends, emotionally, physically, or financially? How have we estranged ourselves from others? What is the effect of our behaviors on ourselves and our relationships?

Treating Others Well Despite the Pain

How have people continued to treat family and friends well, even during the course of their illness? Part of successful management of chronic illness is the attempt to limit its damage to physical damage. People try to leave their relationships intact or even improved during the course of their chronic illness.

Shame and guilt can look similar, but they are very different. A thorough spiritual self-examination looks at what they have done and separates their shame from guilt. The reason for this is that guilt can be useful, while shame is not. Guilt is the moral equivalent of pain. It indicates what's ill or injured and needs to be treated. If someone has an appendicitis, the physical pain will force them to cancel their plans and seek medical care. If they had an appendicitis without physical pain, they would quietly die, but not feel bad. In that sense, the pain is their friend. Similarly, if they felt guilty about their pattern of behavior, they may choose to remove that behavior from their lives.

Shame is not useful. It is a negative, depressing, paralyzing feeling of unworthiness. It tends to keep people stuck. People with chronic illnesses sometimes feel shame about their conditions. There are no circumstances in which shame is actually helpful in treating or caring for the person. There are situations that are embarrassing in chronic illness, but the embarrassment doesn't have to turn to shame.

Guilt versus Shame

Guilt can motivate people towards change, while shame motivates them to judge and condemn themselves. Guilt is about what they do, shame is about who they are. Guilt says, "I made a mistake." Shame says "I am a mistake." Sometimes people who are seriously ill become ashamed of themselves based on the burden that their illness causes for people they care about. "I'm just a burden," they might think or say. The truth is that they are people, not burdens. Their shame leads them to defining themselves as burdens, and their shame makes a difficult situation unbearable.

Sometimes the difference between guilt and shame might seem like splitting hairs, but the hairs are worth splitting because they lead people to opposite conclusions. If a patient is paralyzed due to his drunk driving, then it is a reasonable conclusion that he is guilty of driving drunk and has played a part in causing his injuries. If in fact he has a significant responsibility for his disability then it is reasonable to conclude that he has just as much responsibility for doing the things that lead to well-being, even while paralyzed. However, if he feels shame about his condition, and the part he played in it, he may be as immobilized by shame as he is by his paralysis.

People can feel shame for things that they're not guilty of at all. People tend to feel shame for some things that happen to them. For example, rape victims commonly feel shame, even though they didn't commit the rape. An examination of the shame can lead to the conclusion that the rape victim is not responsible and the shame more appropriately belongs to the perpetrator. Part of the inquiry into the exact nature of their wrongs can include an assessment that they're not wrong at all.

The Twelve Step Opportunity

Twelve Step programs offer an opportunity to turn shame into guilt, guilt into responsibility, responsibility into amends, and amends into freedom. If people feel like bad people, they use Steps Four and Five to identify what's wrong in their lives and to identify those things for which they are guilty. In this they move from being "bad people" to good people who do bad things.

Once people have identified their guilt, they accept responsibility for what they have done, and responsibility for continuing in a process of spiritual growth to become the kind of people who don't do that any more. Out of their sense of responsibility they invite their Higher Power to change them.

As responsible people, living with the guidance and care of their Higher Power, they set out to make amends for what they have done wrong. They bring justice to their lives. When they have done so, they become free.

The Power of Gratitude

The best short inventory of people's spiritual well being is to ask them about gratitude. If they have no gratitude, it means that nothing in their lives is worth being grateful for, and their programs of recovery and spiritual growth need a tune-up. If they can find gratitude, they can usually live in fellowship and harmony with their Higher Power, themselves, and others.

Counting Your Blessings

Gratitude is somewhat of a choice and a spiritual gift. People can make the choice to seek the spiritual gift by noticing what's good in life. A daily gratitude list is a good place to start. The old expression "count your blessings" is practical advice. Many Twelve

Step groups have "gratitude meetings" in which the topic is each person's feelings of and reasons for gratitude. Ultimately, they become grateful for the spiritual benefits of a new, spiritually aware way of life.

A.A. reflects on the gratitude that comes with living the program:

> "Quite as important was the discovery that spiritual principles would solve all my problems. I have since been brought into a way of living infinitely more satisfying and, I hope, more useful than the life I lived before. My old manner of life was by no means a bad one, but I would not exchange its best moments for the worst I have now. I would not go back to it even if I could."[7]

The spiritual principle behind self-examination is courage. It takes courage for people to face themselves, and to write it all down. The hardest part of a written inventory is the beginning. Once people start to write, it often flows from their heart faster than they can record it. While this is a solitary, private exercise, people soon break their isolation by sharing what they have found with God, with themselves, and with another human being. In doing so, they develop integrity.

Suggestions for courage in your life and work:

- Take a searching and fearless moral inventory of yourself, including the categories mentioned in this chapter. Get to know yourself by writing it out.
- Engage your patients in discussing the unexamined areas of their lives, and the ways that what they don't know could be hurting them.
- Encourage them to take on the painful or difficult aspects of their treatment and recovery with courage.
- Encourage patients to use this time of illness for self-examination and reflection.

Bowen F. White

There is no doubt that courage is required on the spiritual path. Perhaps it's even more important for those that don't believe in the concept of the safety net of Mercy. One of the best discussions of courage came from Joseph Campbell, a scholar who studied the mythologies of many different cultures. As an expert in Comparative Mythology, he felt that the Myth of the Grail Guest was the foundation myth of Western culture.

The Grail, in the legend, was the cup passed at the Last Supper or the chalice used to capture the blood of Jesus after he was stabbed in the side with a spear on the cross. Whether or not it exists is controversial. But a myth doesn't rely on facts to convey ideas. As scientists, it is easy to poo poo mythology. Joseph Campbell teaches that a myth is a story about something that never happened. However, it conveys a truth that is happening all the time. It engages the psyche of a culture and then becomes a vehicle to pass culture from generation to generation.

King Arthur and the stories about Knights of the round table are related to this myth. Four different versions of the myth were written between the years 1180–1220 A.D. During this time of the Middle Ages and in medieval Europe, whatever people did with their life was determined by inheritance. If people were born serfs, they begot serfs. If people were born noble, they begot noble people. There was no social mobility. A serf would not find a warm reception if they went up to the castle and said, "I'm tired of living in squalor with the animals. I want to move in with you." Likewise, if a lord went down to the hut and requested asylum from the splendor of nobledom, he would not be well received. The structures of culture were rigid. People did not marry the choice of their heart. They married the choice of their parents. And so on. Whatever they did with their life was determined by their inheritance. That is the background on which the myth unfolds.

In one version of the story the knights are sitting around the round table. The table is round because there is no head of the table. Everyone is of equal stature at the table. Arthur liked to have some sort of adventure before supper. And one night that was provided by the appearance of the Grail. It appeared veiled above the table and Parcival then made a vow to go on a quest after the Holy Grail and find it unveiled.

He did as he said. He went through all manner of travail and much time passed before he finally came to the Grail castle. He was welcomed to the castle and the Grail King was brought forth on a stretcher. The king had been maimed and Parcival was moved by sympathy and compassion to ask the king what ailed him. But, Parcival had been taught that knights don't ask questions. So, he didn't do what was in his own heart and the quest failed. He awoke in the morning and the castle was gone.

But, Parcival, by virtue of his determination continued his quest. And somewhere between 5 and 20 years later, depending on what version you read, he made it back to the Grail castle. This time he allowed what was in his own heart to move him. This second time around, he asked the king what ailed him. And the quest succeeded. The entire kingdom was healed and the knight became a hero.

The knight became a hero by taking a risk. He risked breaking the rules and doing what was in his own heart. Remember, he was taught not to ask any questions. The first time around, he didn't. When given a second chance, he was able to allow sympathy and compassion to move him to break the rules. That was real courage.

The root of the word courage is "coeur," which means heart in French. The definition of hero is the one who follows the path of courage. When people do what has heart, meaning, and passion for them, they do what is not only best for them, but what is also best for the common good.

Courage is required to break the rules of people's own conditioning, their own inheritance, and to do what is in their hearts. They inherit certain cultural biases that set them up to be focused upon doing the will of others. They learn to be externally referenced, tuned into the needs of others while learning to be internally neglectful. That is what good people do. To be that concerned with getting their own needs met is to be selfish. And how can they be selfish yet still be a good person?

■ **LITERAL TRANSLATION OF THE BIBLE**

Wisdom might be found in the Bible. Although some people take the Bible literally, I don't. Others don't take any of it as the truth, I do. Even for non-believers, most would admit that it contains some good stories and lessons for living a values-centered life.

■ **BIBLICAL COURAGE STORIES**

The Bible provides stories of courage. Two examples follow. There is this story of Moses who leads his people out of bondage in Egypt. They begin their journey to the promised land by wandering around—for 40 years. This might be where Jewish humor comes from. "Moses, I don't want to seem impolite, but are you sure you are talking to the right guy?" Let's face it, a sense of humor would be necessary to sustain someone for 40 wandering-around years. Early into the journey, Moses left abruptly for a mountain retreat. He was not doing what others in his community were telling him to do. He did, rather, what his heart told him to do. He went up Mt. Siani, the site of the retreat and came back with the boon, the gift to the community.

Now, while he was gone, the rest of his flock took advantage of the opportunity and had a huge drunken party. There were probably some folks who didn't go along with this behavior. They were probably scolding Moses in absentia for his irresponsible neglect of the tribe. It probably went something like this, "Can you believe that Moses? Taking off for forty days while we are left here to our own debauchery. How selfish." Moses had the courage of his convictions and followed the direction of his heartfelt guidance. In so doing he was able to garner for the whole community the gift of the Ten Commandments. When he returned he discovered just how desperately they were needed.

If people are willing to live their lives from the heart, to have the courage to live from the inside out, other people may see them as troublemakers. Matthew 21:12–15 tells of a rule breaker that lived life courageously. He did not go along with the status quo and would not nod to the authority figures of his own religion. He healed people on the Sabbath, the day of rest. He disturbed the commerce of the money changers in the temple. His behavior put him in harm's way.

That Rabbi had an amazing ability to heal, on any day. In fact, after he began his healing ministry he returned the sight of the blind, made lame people walk and even raised people from the dead. Miraculous stories of healing abounded. His healing gift came after he left his followers for a 40-day desert retreat. It was upon his return that he began healing individuals and later the community.

But it's not difficult to imagine what people in the community said when they found out that the Rabbi had abandoned them. "Here I've come all this way with him and he goes off by himself. How could he leave us like this? We came to be with him and he wants to be alone. What do you mean, he's gone into the desert alone? We need him here. The suffering is here. How selfish of him to leave us like this."

By doing what was in his heart, he offended not only the authority figures of his own church, but others in his community. However, by following the lead of his heart, his courage still speaks to us across the ages. For he returned from the desert to give his gift. And that gift provides healing for the whole community.

■ FOLLOWING THE PATH OF THE HEART

We live in a Judeo-Christian culture. But the values that we are discussing are ubiquitous in all religions or at least in the lives of the founding figures of those religions. And their advice to us is inclusive of following the path of the heart. Just like the Grail Quest for the West, the wisdom literature of the planet supports courage as a central tenet of the spiritual path.

But for me to have the courage to follow that path, I really need encouragement. I need other people in my life to give me their support when I lose heart. Those are relationships that sustain me on the spiritual journey. Our patients, whether chronically ill or not, also need that kind of support to do what is in their own hearts. Clinicians, family and friends may oppose certain activities of the infirm because of some medical condition. Why? Because we feel we know what's best for them. This isn't always the case.

The Importance of Play Cannot Be Overemphasized

O. Fred Donaldson, Ph.D., wrote a book called *Playing by Heart: The Vision and Practice of Belonging*.[8] It is now being self-published by the organization, Touch the Future Foundation, located in Los Angeles, CA. Donaldson is a "play" specialist. In his book, Fred tells the story of a child named Paul. "This kindergartner had leukemia and his parents were afraid that physical play would hasten his death." His parents felt they knew best. The story goes, "One day Paul came to me and asked if I would invite his parents to school for a meeting. The following afternoon the four of us met in the classroom. Paul began quietly, "I want to play with Fred. I know that I am not going to live as long as the three of you, but I want to live as if I were." His sincerity was powerful. There were tears in our eyes as all agreed that he could play. When he came to school the following day he was so excited and he played so fully that he was exhausted and had to stay home and rest the next day. The pattern of coming to school for a morning and resting the next continued. About a month later, Paul died of leukemia."

Paul was 5 years old at the time of his death. He had not yet finished kindergarten yet he was in touch with what was important in life. He knew his own heart, was in touch with the risks involved in following its lead, and played with Fred. That is true courage, and his parents gave permission because they understood that their son deserved to have what was in his heart, even if it broke theirs. That is courage also.

Death is not the enemy. It's the inevitable. The question is, can people live with the courage of a 5-year-old boy and play with life? And can they help their patients, their playmates, do the same? "Unless you become like little children, you will never enter the Kingdom of Heaven" (Matthew 18:30).

Ways in which you might encourage courage in your chronically ill patient include:

- Take the time to discover what has heart/meaning/passion for the patient.
- If they don't know, help them to discover what is that thing has the most heart for them? Ask them, "What is it they'd like to do, but never had the courage to do before?"
- Ask your patients if there are any family members/acquaintances with whom they'd like to reconcile?
- Encourage your patients to take risks in their personal lives, much like an entrepreneur does in the business world each and every day.

REFERENCES

1. *Alcoholics Anonymous*, p. 66.
2. Ibid., p. 58.
3. Ibid., pp. 67–68.
4. Ibid., p. 68.
5. Ibid., p. 69.
6. Ibid., p. 82.
7. Ibid., p. 43.
8. O. Fred Donaldson, *Playing by Heart: The Vision and Practice of Belonging*, Health Communications, Inc., 1993.

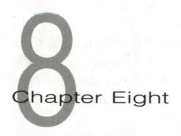

Chapter Eight

Principle 5: Integrity

John A. Mac Dougall

> Knowing others is intelligence;
> knowing yourself is true wisdom.
> Mastering others is strength;
> mastering yourself is true power.
>
> If you realize that you have enough,
> you are truly rich.
> If you stay in the center
>
> and embrace death with your whole heart,
> you will endure forever.
>
> *Tao Te Ching*[1]

Step Five and the Integrity Principle

Step Five states: "Admitted to God, to ourselves, and to another human being the exact nature of our wrongs."

■ INTEGRITY FOUND ONLY AFTER OWNING SHAME AND GUILT

If people have the courage to do a thorough self-examination of their spirit and character, and keep the results to themselves, spiritual progress stops there. A sense of shame may keep them stuck in their spiritual development. Their fears about losing face and fears about change seem like reasons to keep the discreditable parts of themselves hidden. They might maintain a pattern of denial in the hope that denial will bring their comfort level back. However, once they know the truth about their character and conduct, they will be restless, irritable, and discontent until something is done.

Their examination of conscience has helped to turn their shame into guilt. Instead of feeling badly about who they are, they now have identified what they have done wrong. They have hopefully resolved not to repeat those wrongs. In order to make their resolutions come true, they need to open up to their Higher Power, their conscious selves, and to at least one other person. They need to take responsibility for who they are, what they've done, and what they have become. By owning their shameful and guilty aspects, they develop integrity.

■ SPIRITUAL GROWTH IS THE RESULT OF STEP FIVE

The Fifth Step of the Twelve Step programs reads, "We admitted to God, to ourselves, and to another human being the exact nature of our wrongs." This step, like most, makes no mention of alcohol or drugs. It is for spiritual growth. There are two major definitions of integrity. The first is: "The condition of having no part or element taken away or wanting; undivided or unbroken state; material wholeness, completeness, entirety."[2]

■ ADAPTABILITY AND CHRONIC ILLNESS

The chronic illness patient may find this definition of integrity irritating, thinking that only the physically intact and well person can have this kind of integrity. Becoming whole while ill or injured involves seeing themselves as complete just the way they are. In any area of disability, people develop a compensation somewhere in their bodies or in their ways of life. People who are injured by strokes do retraining of the brain so that uninjured parts carry on for the damaged parts. Diabetics find enjoyment in the parts of the food chain that are both safe and pleasurable. Recovering alcoholics learn to enjoy sobriety. People with terminal illnesses develop the ability to get great intensity out of life each day and find ways to leave lasting legacies. Humans are adaptable.

■ A SENSE OF GRATITUDE FOR LIFE

In 1972, I was doing Clinical Pastoral Education at Bellevue Hospital and New York University Medical Center. One of the patients, Roy Campanella, was a famous catcher for the Brooklyn Dodgers. He was paralyzed from the waist down from a car accident in the 1950s. He came into the hospital a couple of times a year to be treated for circulatory problems. He was tied to a pallet, which was suspended in a circular frame. By being in this contraption, he could be rotated like clock hands to shift his blood flow. He was still known among New Yorkers as a famous baseball player. He would have himself wheeled around the hospital to visit the sick and injured there. He was a cheerful gentleman, who spent extra time on the orthopedics ward with people who had major injuries.

As a chaplain trainee, I was supposed to bring him some spiritual benefit. However, he benefited me much more by sharing his warm, loving spirit and his sense of gratitude for life. He was free of resentments and self-pity. Today, I read in the sports pages the stories of millionaire crybabies who are stuck in resentment and self-pity for not being the highest paid player or being the most famous. I firmly believe that Roy Campanella had much more integrity than many of today's uninjured athletes.

■ BEING SEEN AS LESS THAN WHOLE

The nature of illness or injury is that some part of the person seems taken away. People beg in to see themselves with physical limitations, rather than as a whole person. There are suddenly things they can't do, or can only do with difficulty.

■ BUSY BEING SICK

When flu swept Hazelden many of the staff couldn't come in to work because they were busy being sick. Being kept away from work was shocking to some because they hadn't been that sick before. They adapted to the short term problem by staying home. If it were a long term illness, they would need other adaptations.

■ A CHANGING WORKPLACE

Some people with chronic illness have started to work at home by "telecommuting" via computer, phone, and fax. Some prisoners work as airline reservations agents by answering the airline's from prison workrooms. Their limitations are imposed by the state rather than by illness, but the customers have no way of knowing whether the agent they were talking to was telecommuting from home due to disability or telecommuting from prison due to necessity.

People with limited mobility get handicapped license plates, specially equipped vans, and powered wheelchairs to restore their ability to get around. People dependent on oxygen, insulin, or who require emergency bee sting shots carry portable supplies. Others with mental retardation have assisted living situations and job coaches to restore the ability to function in society. Alcoholics and addicts get sponsors, home groups, and programs of recovery to rehabilitate and learn sober living skills.

■ ATTITUDE MAKES ALL THE DIFFERENCE

Attitude makes the difference between being broken and having integrity. I have just turned 50 years old. Some people regard turning 50 as a disaster and treat it like a chronic illness. Some people offer sympathy on the occasion of getting older, as the number four turns to five on the imaginary odometer of life. I'm not troubled by turning 50. In fact, I like the idea. After all, I've considered the alternative: not turning 50. The only way to avoid turning 50 is to die by 49. Compared to that, turning 50 seems like a good deal. I hope I turn 60, 70, even 80!

■ ATTITUDE IS EVERYTHING

I have a bad headache on the average of once every 10 days. I have no choice about the headaches, but I have a choice of my attitude about them. I can be angry and find people to be angry at. Years ago, there was a television ad for an analgesic in which a mother was being hostile to her adult daughter. The daughter's line was, "Mother, please! Sure you have a headache, but don't take it out on me!" The pain remedy was offered as treatment for both headache and hurt feelings. Another remedy for hurt feelings would be the willingness to have a literal headache without giving others figurative headaches.

Occasionally guests have arrived at my home while I am lying down on the couch with a cloth blindfold to block the light. They've routinely apologized for coming over when I had headaches, as if they were responsible for my pain. They would offer to go away because I was sick. My attitude was that my headaches would do the minimum damage to my choices and so they were welcome to stay. Sometimes I passed up dinner, but my guests were welcome to remain and eat with my wife. My attitude of keeping my pain to myself has helped my relationship with my wife too. If I passed on my pain in the form of hostility and contempt, I'd be divorced by now. As it is, she appreciates me more because I don't inflict distress on her.

■ COPING IS EASIER WITH A POSITIVE ATTITUDE

A positive attitude helps people cope with mental illnesses, as well. Antidepressant drugs are a blessing when they work, but they don't work for everyone, and they don't work right away. William Glasser's "Reality Therapy" consists of a set of positive attitudes and actions that get us unstuck. Rational Emotive Therapy states that feelings are not caused by events. Rather, they are caused by events that are filtered through attitudes. Feelings are based less on the triggering events than on the attitudes that people have about those events.

■ SUCCESSFULLY ADAPTING TO LIFE

At a Twelve Step meeting for incest survivors, one woman who had multiple personalities was speaking. She said, "I'm sick of my therapist calling me 'a multiple' as if that were an insult. So I've started calling him 'a single'. The poor guy, when he's alone, he has no one to talk to."

Alan D. added, "I know some people who have less than one personality. We can call them partials." The group laughed. This has nothing to do with curing the woman's mental illness, but it has everything to do with finding a successful adaptation to her life as it exists in the present.

■ DEFINING A CRISIS

When I was a trainee at Hazelden, one of my frequent comments was, "That's not a crisis." Finally, one of the supervisors asked me what I would consider to be a crisis. I said, "If a patient is out walking on the thin ice on the lake, and they haven't fallen through, it's a problem. If they have fallen through and drowned, it's a tragedy. If they have fallen through and they haven't drowned yet, it's a crisis." That narrow definition of a crisis helps keep me from being in a crisis mode very often. If our attitude is one of perpetual crisis, our bodies ultimately will pay the price.

On Wednesday mornings I speak in Hazelden's Family Program on Spirituality and Recovery. I am not a morning person. But, I have come to learn that the attitude you choose in the morning affects your entire day. My perspective is that it's really night everywhere, but the sun is on fire. Rarely do I feel like giving an hour lecture in the morning. If I get out of bed and say, "Oh, shit!" then that's what I will get all day. If my attitude is more like "I don't want to do this" it will become a long hour for everyone. Instead, I deliberately choose an attitude of energy and enthusiasm. This carries me through the hour and is contagious too. Listeners often become energetic and enthusiastic, as well. This is not a false front or show, but a choice to orient in a positive direction. Once I have begun to choose enthusiasm, it becomes real.

■ RESTORING VIRTUE

Integrity is also defined as: "Soundness of moral principle; the character of uncorrupted virtue, esp. in relation to truth and fair dealing; uprightness, honesty, sincerity."[2] It may be too late in life for uncorrupted virtue, but by people admitting their exact nature of their wrongs, they set the stage for their restoration of virtue.

Just as people need to accept their physical brokenness and limitations, they need to accept the brokenness in their conduct so far. Pretense is bad. It isn't possible to get real joy out of a false life. People instinctively dislike the hypocrite because they can sense that they are not well. Bank robber Willie Sutton is admired for saying that he robbed banks because that's where the money is. He isn't admired for robbing banks, but rather for being frank and open about his motivations. Integrity is inherently attractive.

People begin the process of restoring their character by admitting what's wrong with them. The process of admitting is likely to be accompanied by a temporary rise in anxiety. This is more than offset by the sense of relief that follows. Admitting what's wrong isn't a quick fix, but rather the beginning of a process of restoration.

■ THE IMPORTANCE OF COMPASSIONATE LISTENERS

People need to admit in an atmosphere of compassion. They need to have an understanding of a compassionate Higher Power. If they envision an angry God, their admission will be far from complete. If they have developed hope and faith in their Higher Power relationship they will have the courage to face the God of their understanding. They need a compassionate listener. Clergy have traditionally filled this role, but anyone who will keep their confidences and deal with them in a loving way will do. People in Twelve Step programs often do their admitting with a sponsor, who is likely to have many of the same wrongs. They need to be compassionate with themselves in this process. They have a common humanity with their listener, and they are beloved children of their Higher Power. When people are listened to and loved, they can finally be free to speak the truth about their lives. The people chosen to hear their stories need to have compassion for them just the way they are, not the way they will be when their soundness of moral principle is restored. These confidants need enough integrity of their own to respect the person's confidentiality, and a clear enough moral vision to remind others of the exact nature of their wrongs, instead of getting mired in detail.

■ THE BENEFITS OF TELLING THE TRUTH

Clinicians can benefit from this truth telling and restoration of integrity to improve their spirituality and their art of clinical practice. When there are discreditable elements in their professional lives, they weigh on both the skill and the grace with which people carry out their work. To be consistent, whole, and complete in their practice, clinicians may want to have a trusted peer or peer group provide clinical supervision. This supervision can be on the spirit in which they carry out their work, as well as the practical standards they are upholding. Their clinical practice can have the "truth and fair dealing, uprightness, honesty, and sincerity" that defines integrity.

For both the clinician and the patient integrity involves consistency and congruency. The thoughts, words, and actions can then flow seamlessly. What people say or do usually reveals what that person is thinking. People think, speak, and act from their spiritual centers. This is somewhat harder for a woman who has been socialized to take care of the feelings of others. If she is finely attuned to her partner and children, she may tune out her own self. First her actions, then her words, and ultimately even her thoughts may be reflections of other people. For her, integrity means finding her own authentic voice. Telling the truth about people's lives doesn't automatically restore soundness of moral principle. For the restoration to be complete, people need willingness, humility, compassion, justice, perseverance, spiritual awareness, and service. Everyone, especially patients with a chronic illness should make a special effort to practice integrity in their everyday lives as this can make a real difference in their well being.

Suggestions for integrity in your life and work:

- Admit to God, to yourself, and one other human being the exact nature of your wrongs.
- Consider having a clinical sponsor, with whom you discuss your own spirituality and how that impacts your work.
- Give your patients the opportunity to unburden themselves about what's wrong in their lives.
- Give your patients the opportunity to be sick, cranky, despairing, and all the things that "good" patients don't want to be.
- Treat every single human being that you meet with dignity and respect, not because of who they are, but because of who you are.

Bowen F. White

. . . Go start some huge foolish project like Noah,
It makes absolutely no difference what people think of you.

Rumi

Integrity is a word we hear bandied around all the time. It is defined
as an adherence to a code of values. Companies usually include
the word in their corporate values. It gets plenty of lip service, but
is often in short supply. A synonym for integrity is honesty. It has
already been established that the concept of "honesty is the best
policy" is rarely followed.

The spiritual path requires both integrity and honesty as knot
material. The root of the word "integrity" goes back through
Middle English, Old French, and Latin. It is derived from older
words that meant completeness, purity, and whole. It is taking the
risk for people to admit that they make mistakes every day.
People risk being vulnerable by acting with integrity. It is the showing of what is going on inside to the outside world. Instead of being
who they think other people want them to be, they are who they
want to be. People take the risk of being who they are even if it dis-
appoints other people. Risks are definitely involved.

When someone has integrity they are congruent. In other
words, what is going on inside the person, their beliefs, thoughts,
and feelings are expressed in their words and actions. What they
do is in alignment with their thinking and feeling. That is integrity.
It is all too rare in a culture where people learn to be incongruent
to survive. They repress how they really think and feel while
expressing only what is safe to say. That is incongruent.

By acting with integrity, people risk exposure to the bullets of
ridicule and rejection. When they box up their opinions for expression at a later, safer date, they can slide along with the dominant
culture and avoid being cannon fodder. To act with integrity
requires trust because they become much more vulnerable. That
trust may be in the quality of relationship that they have with an

individual, group or God. And/or that trust may be in knowing themselves and knowing that being phony is no longer something they choose to do.

Authentic expression is one way to be a real person. Young children are good at authentic expression. Their exuberance, spontaneity, playfulness, curiosity, laughter, and tears are immediately apparent. They are pure in that what is shown on the outside is an expression of what is going on inside. That kind of purity is also reached by people who are able to break free of the fetters of cultural conditioning. Something happens and they realize that they hold the key to open the door of the prison house of cultural conditioning into a free future.

The chronically ill often experience this. When they become sick they are given a license to drop their guises that they used to hide behind and step out into the light. While dropping their old concerns for the superficial they become what some would call alarmingly straight forward. An OB-GYN from Maine, Christiane Northrup, recalls that some women with PMS state that that is the time of the month when they actually say what is on their minds. Although other people may not like what they hear, it is the truth. Those with PMS may bottle up their emotions the rest of the month, but when the lid comes off, the truth erupts.

It is a sad commentary on today's culture. What is it that makes people so reticent to be real, that they have to wait for some hormonal imbalance, illness, job loss, or other loss to live a life of integrity?

■ A GIRL NAMED SUE

In ninth grade, I had a girlfriend named Sue. We had a great relationship. We both loved to dance and we could kiss for hours without coming up for air. Things were going well until my birthday. At this time she gave me a card that caused me to break up with her. I didn't know why. But, I knew that I had no choice but to break up with Sue. Virginia Satir, an authority in the field of family therapy, said that our ability to see choices is directly related to self-esteem. My ninth grade girlfriend's birthday card to me was very positive and expressed her caring feelings to me. Yet, I had no choice but to break up with Sue. I didn't know why at that time. However, I did figure it out at our 25th high school reunion. I approached Sue with my revelation.

"Sue, how do you do?" I inquired.

"Fine," she replied.

"Do you remember when I broke up with you in high school?" I asked.

"Yes," she replied promptly.

"I know why I did it," I announced.

"Let's hear it," she said.

"I broke up with you not because of how I felt about you. I broke up with you because of how I felt about me. I did it because I felt like a piece of shit. If you got too close, you might get a whiff. If you got too close you'd know my secret, that I wasn't worth knowing. I pushed you away to stay safe. I'm sorry."

She understood that immediately. This kind of thinking isn't all that uncommon. I think that we all have a secret that we share that we don't want anyone to know about. I call it our best kept secret. And that secret is that we all have feelings of inadequacy but we do not want anyone else to find out. So, we walk around acting like we know what we're doing so no one discovers our secret.

I've learned to be ashamed of myself. Even though we can be quite good at task specific behaviors, even though we know how to do a lot of things well, it doesn't make those feelings of shame go away. So we don't feel very good about ourselves and therefore have problems with, among other things, integrity.

■ FEELING INADEQUATE

When clinicians are not sure what to say to a patient, do they say, "I don't know what to say?" Or, do they say something because they feel that they are supposed to know? When it feels as if they are not able to do much to help a suffering person and they are feeling very inadequate, do they admit that they feel inadequate? Or do they concoct some "new" intervention from the fountain of innovative remedies?

To a chronically ill patient, it may be useful to cut the bullshit. Patients don't want to be patronized. When people are sick, wouldn't they want the integrity of their doctor to be apparent? Being frightened can get in the way of this kind of authenticity. People can't pretend that they aren't afraid. Well, they can pretend, but they have to be able to attend to the suffering among them in spite of those feelings. Because clinicians have feelings of inadequacy doesn't mean that they are inadequate. Look at all people have accomplished to be able to serve the infirm. By owning that those feelings are present, they can shine the flashlight of their attention on that part of them and the energy will flow in that direction. They can then get their own egocentric concerns out of the way so they can seek the help they need to best tend those given them to serve.

That might mean consulting another doctor or another practitioner. Or it might mean asking for help from the Great Physician, alone or in the presence of the chronically ill person. It might even mean sharing the fact that the clinician is sorry that they are not able to provide more relief to the suffering person in their care.

That kind of behavior may not be normal, standard of care medicine. But, it would go a long way toward the establishment of a relationship of integrity. And in that kind of reality-based relationship, healing is a mutual experience.

If clinicians say they don't know why something is happening, will their patients' opinion of them be diminished? Perhaps that's a risk. What is more likely is the reverse. Patients will see that their clinicians are like them. That connection with the patient and the clinician allows the patient to risk more. And in that authentic dialogue, God can show up. Then, there's healing all around.

Chuck Hogan, a bright, insightful teacher with a great sense of humor is, among other things, a coach of professional golfers on the LPGA tour as well as executives who aspire to improve their game. He talks about how executives, who are running billion dollar companies, pay him thousands of dollars to teach them not to shake standing over a three foot putt. The cause of their trepidation is not that they may miss the putt. Rather, it is how they will be perceived should they miss the short putt.

Isn't that what keeps people from being congruent? Their concern about the opinions of others gets in the way and causes them to be anxious over their metaphorical three foot putts. They obsess about their image in the eyes of others and integrity goes in the toilet. And the culture feeds the obsession.

Madison Avenue shows people images and delivers messages that promote feelings of inadequacy. Secret inadequate feelings get reinforced over and over and over. People then purchase products and perform behaviors that compensate. If people wear certain clothes, drive certain cars, take certain vacations, send their children to certain schools, live in certain neighborhoods with well landscaped yards, etc., then people will not merely see them as adequate, but superior. Isn't that what people want, for others to see them as superior, on top of their game?

People complain about politicians that make decisions by opinion polls. They complain about the politicians' lack of integrity, saying one thing now and another later, to justify their vote. But they are a reflection of people's collective consciousness. They are reflecting back to us, ourselves. They avoid the risk of going against the grain because they want to be re-elected. They want to win the vote. The end justifies the means. We do the same thing. For what office are we running? Aren't we continually taking polls to see which way the local political winds are blowing?

We are so concerned with how we are perceived by others that we get distracted and thrown off balance. We are busy focusing on trying to be adequate for person "A." So for person "A" we are A. But, for person "B" we need to be adequate too. So for person "B" we are B. For person "C" we need to be seen as adequate also. For "C" we are C. For an alphabet of people in our outer life, we are an alphabet of people in our inner life. It is stressful because you have to be constantly on your toes. It eats energy and drains it out of the psyche.

It is much less stressful being one person for all people. It requires less energy to be congruent, to be a person of integrity. Perhaps it is because at those times we are complete, wholly who we are. We can relax into just being ourselves. That is freedom. And by us being who we are, real with our patients, they can be who they really are with us. Let the healing begin.

Ways in which you might encourage your chronically ill patients to incorporate integrity in their lives:

- Encourage your patients to express instead of repress how they think and feel.
- Be open and honest with your patients. You cannot have integrity without honesty.
- Act with integrity. Remember that the best moral decision is the best decision. Act with integrity in all aspects of your life. Encourage your patients to do the same.
- Have relationships with other people that help you remember to act with integrity when you feel the price is too high. Encourage your patients to do the same.

REFERENCES

1. S. Mitchell, *Tao Te Ching, A New English Version*, Harper Collins, New York, 1992, p. 33.
2. *Oxford English Dictionary*, 2nd edn., Oxford University Press, 1993.

Chapter Nine

Principle 6: Willingness

John A. Mac Dougall

> When you have faults, do not fear to abandon them.
> *The Confucian Analects*, book 1:8

Step Six and the Willingness Principle

Step Six states: "Were entirely ready to have God remove all these defects of character."

The Art of Change

It is good when people admit their wrongs. Changing them, however, is even better. A simple but misleading decision at this point would be for people to make a decision to change the behavior themselves. People often decide to change themselves, without noticing that chronic illnesses do not respond well to self-will. Self-help will not do. People grow spiritually within a network of relationships: with a Higher Power, with themselves, and with other people. Self-reliance is valuable. Democracy, economic growth, freedom of speech, and thought all benefit from the efforts of self-reliant individuals. Self-reliance also has limits. It becomes

167

a problem when people begin to believe that they can handle anything by themselves.

Interdependence is a Good Thing

The reality of people's everyday lives illustrates that they are more interdependent than independent. Few people weave their own clothes, grow their own food, distill their own gasoline, create their own pharmaceuticals and render their own medical care. When major life tasks arise such as spiritual growth or the management of chronic illness, suddenly people act as if they could handle it themselves. The more successful they become at managing their own lives, the more shocking it is when there are aspects of their lives that are unmanageable.

To grow spiritually, and have loving relationships with a Higher Power, with themselves, and with other human beings, people need to become willing to be cared for and healed by their Higher Power. Care and healing can be physical, mental, emotional, spiritual, or any combination of these factors. In order for their Higher Power to care for them, they need to be willing to accept that care.

■ **A HEALING STORY**

One of the healing stories of Jesus illustrates the difficulty they can have in becoming willing to be changed by a Higher Power.

"Now in Jerusalem by the Sheep Gate there is a pool, called in Hebrew Beth-zatha, which has five porticoes. In these lay many invalids—blind, lame, and paralyzed, waiting for the stirring of the water; for an angel of the Lord went down at certain seasons into the pool, and stirred up the water; whoever stepped in first after the stirring of the water was made well from whatever disease that person had. One man was there who had been ill for 38 years. When Jesus saw him lying there and knew that he had been there a long time, he said to him, 'Do you want to be made well?' "[1]

What a cruel question! Of course he wanted to be made well. Wouldn't anyone? Not necessarily. We can become used to and comfortable with our illnesses, be they physical, mental, emotional, or spiritual. They can have secondary gains that we don't want to lose. Instead of saying yes, the man who had been lying there for 38 years came up with an excuse why he was never the first one in the pool: "Sir, I have no one to put me into the pool when the water is stirred up; and while I am making my way, someone else steps down ahead of me."[2]

His excuse is a stand-in for the truth. The truth is that he wasn't ready to have God remove his illness. If he had wanted, he could have laid at the edge of the pool, and just rolled into it when the water first stirred. Jesus didn't respond to his excuse at all, he just healed the man, even though the man didn't ask for healing. In truth, that's just what we're afraid of.

It Cannot Happen Without Willingness

To become ready, people need willingness to have God remove their defects of character.

People have many reasons why they haven't changed. They may like their character defects. They may believe that their defects are what provides their lives with color and texture. Without their character defects, they imagine, they'd be bland and uninteresting.

■ **REMOVING CHARACTER DEFECTS**

My birthplace is New York City. I used to say that without my character defects, I'd be in danger of having no character at all. I imagined that my rudeness was simply a natural expression of being a New Yorker. Once I admitted this particular defect of character, and became willing to have God remove it, the process was underway to leave it behind. I am much less rude than I used to be, and still feel very much a New Yorker.

Protection Against Pain

People may be using their character defects as defenses against pain. A habit of reflexive lying defends them against the pain of the truth. Children who grow up in a hostile or critical environment learn that the safest answer to any question is, "I don't know." For example: When mom asks, "Who took the cookies?" their standard reply will always be, "I don't know." If asked what they would like to do on the weekend, these children learn that the wrong answer leads to pain, so once again they learn to answer, "I don't know" even when they do. Over time, they forget that they know the answers to many of life's questions and automatically reply "I don't know." In reality, they are ignoring what they think and feel. Alcoholics and addicts lie about their addictions rather than face the pain of knowing their lives are out of control, or the pain of giving up the drug that appears to be comforting them. Political leaders lie, mislead, and "spin" their actions rather than face the pain of opposition from constituents. The character defect of lying takes on the function of protection against pain.

An oppositional nature defends people against the pain of change. Employees sometimes take on an automatic opposition to anything that is changing, to defend against the pain of insecurity. They can be seen mourning the days of lifetime employment. Rather than conforming to the changing conditions in the workplace and facing the painful possibility of not keeping up, they dig in, opposing and criticizing anything new without even examining it. This may feel like protection against becoming unable to do their jobs, but actually it makes job loss more likely.

Greed appears to treat the anxiety of economic insecurity. Struggling for any economic advantage feels like behavior that leads to safety, but it leads into a competition in which no amount of money is ever enough.

Gossip: A Signal of Untrustworthiness

Gossip defends against loneliness. Gossip is a way of being connected to others. The gossip is connected briefly to the listeners, and the gossip feels like a connection with the person being gossiped about. In reality, it creates distance rather than closeness and trust, because it signals the gossip's untrustworthiness. Hostility and contempt for others defends against the fear of intimacy. If people keep finding fault with everyone, then others will keep their distance and in turn those who gossip are "safe" from the possibility that they will become close with others.

Women may already have experienced a lot of willingness, but it is often willingness to cooperate with other people, and willingness to help them. Many are willing to defer to the ideas of their fathers or husbands, but less willing to be reliant on their own sense of what is right. Often their willingness does not extend to a willingness to rely on a Higher Power and a program of personal growth for their own healing.

The goal of this phase of spiritual development is to become willing to have their Higher Power change them, not to change themselves. A natural choice is to try to quickly fix defects, rather than opening up to the slower and more profound change of spiritual growth. If people try to just "not do it any more" without a change of heart, they just dig themselves into a deeper hole. For example, if they identify bad tempers as problems, then a logical choice is to decide to simply hold their tempers, and not blow up at people. The problem is that their spirit remains unchanged. They're trying to change behavior without being changed at heart. The stress of holding their tempers can add to the size of the next explosion when their control ultimately slips.

Making Amends

When people try to make amends for their behavior without having the underlying character change that goes along with it, their amends end up being fresh offenses. If they have the character defect of argumentativeness, they may make apologies, but then they are likely to go on to state why they were right all along. Thus they repeat the original offenses, even when trying to fix things. If their defect is jealousy, they may apologize for jealous outbursts, and then go on to inquire further, revealing that the jealousy is still there.

■ SPIRITUAL PROGRESS

Living with character defects is the easier, softer way. People have grown accustomed and comfortable with them. They make people who they are. They defend against pain and guide others to keep a safe distance from them. Living without character defects is more satisfying. Without them, people no longer have to live at a distance from their Higher Power, themselves, and others. To make spiritual progress, people need to open themselves to the deep internal changes that can only be brought about by a loving God.

Suggestions for willingness in your life and work:

- Become entirely ready to have God remove all your defects of character.
- Be willing to learn and grow, by studying methods other than your own, being open minded to those that seem foolish.
- Be willing to learn and grow by listening to your patients. Your knowledge about their diseases is different than their knowledge of their illnesses.
- Encourage your patients to be willing to learn and grow as a result of their illness.

Bowen F. White

> The human heart can go to the lengths of God
> Dark and cold we may be, but this is no winter now
> The frozen miseries of centuries breaks cracks begins to move
> The thunder is the thunder of the floes, the thaw, the flood, the
>   upstart Spring
> Thank God our time is now when wrong comes up to face us
>   everywhere
> Never to leave us till we take the longest stride of soul men
>   ever took
> Affairs are now soul size
> The enterprise is exploration into God
> What are we waiting for?
> It takes so many thousand years to wake.
> Will we wake for pity's sake?
>
> Christopher Fry, *A Sleep of Prisoners*

The poem speaks volumes. It shows that the human heart can go to the lengths of God. It is possible. "Can" is the key word. As humans, people can with their very human hearts go there. It is possible. But will they? Will they be willing to do this thing that they can do, that is possible for them to do?

It is interesting to see how people use language. People often say the word "can't" when they mean "won't." When someone says that they can't do something it is as if they are not able. In fact, that only means that they won't. They are unwilling to do something. People are unwilling, at the moment, to change the course of their lives to do what they can. They put it off until later. Then something happens to them and that thing that was a possibility moves into the light of their attention. And energy flows in that direction, toward what they had put off.

The poem states, "Thank God our time is now when wrong comes up to face us everywhere ..." Perhaps it is their time now, the now that they experience when they have their world stopped by wrong looking them in the face. The innocent face of the patient with a genetic disorder or some other malady that they had no part in creating or the still innocent face of the patient that made choices that resulted in their infirmity, those who see themselves as a wrong person looking back in the mirror of their illness. For everyone, the time is now. People have all done wrong, been wrong, been wronged and thought wrong enough to have earned the right to have this now-God time. Why put it off any longer? The alarm is ringing. It's a new day and the friend is at the door, "Can you come out to play today?" People may know they can, but will they? That is the real question.

The poem states, "Will we wake..." Yes, but the question is, when? For most mortals that is usually when they reach some very firm footing. Some call that firmness a bottom. People fall off their high horse and land often on their bottom. That ground is the fertile soil of the new, promised land. It may not smell promising. They may think it stinks. But, what they may be smelling is the fertilizer for their own growth.

■ ACTING ON MY WILL

This personal story demonstrates the act of will quite nicely. It shows how by acting on my will instead of someone else's, there were very different consequences. When I was 23 years old, I took off on a great adventure. I was a college graduate and had the military behind me. For three years I had dreamed of taking off and traveling the world. When I landed in New York on my way to Europe, my buddy and traveling companion left a message at the Swiss Air counter that he would not be arriving until the next day.

I had $1,200, a backpack, sleeping bag and a roundtrip ticket to Geneva. I did not have a hotel room in New York or a willingness to dump any of my limited financial resources there. I boarded the plane for Europe. That was an act of will. My will.

While on board the transatlantic flight, I had to be willing to consider some new possibilities. One, that I might not see my friend and would therefore be traveling alone. That was a little worrisome. I noticed that the plane made a stop in Lisbon, Portugal. Although I didn't know what I would do there, I decided to disembark. That was another act of will.

Over the next several days I decided to go south instead of east. That choice would take me into Africa across the Straits of Gibraltar and into a warmer winter climate. One month later, I was alone in North Africa in the town of Marrekech, Morocco. I was depressed. I couldn't figure it out since I was finally doing what I dreamed of doing for over three years. I suspected that I was depressed because I was in a foreign country where they talked a foreign language and ate strange food. The environment was different. The religion was unfamiliar. There was nothing familiar there to hold on to. I was adrift in a sea of uncertainty. I experienced that loss, that sense of isolation and loneliness as depression.

When I examined it closely it was clear to me that the only thing I knew for sure was that I didn't know anything. I was a college graduate, 23 years old and completely ignorant. I knew what other people had said, what other people had written. But, the only thing that I personally knew was that I didn't know anything.

This was a huge "Ah Ha" experience for me. A light bulb went off when I saw my obvious ignorance. I figured that if I didn't know anything, that was a very firm foundation on which to build my house of self. That structure would be built one brick at a time, experiential brick by experiential brick. If I didn't know anything, then anyone could be my teacher. But, I would test what they said to see if it were true for me by virtue of my experience.

Simultaneously with the above realization, my world began to open up. I quit thinking about doing something so I could then tell my friends about it on my return. I saw the new, unfamiliar world around me as a place to learn. A real sense of adventure replaced the depressed perspective that had dominated my initial emotional tone.

I also realized that this experience was a blessing that would not have been possible had my buddy been there. Without him there to mirror back to me a familiar, albeit culturally biased, ethos, I had to confront the fact that I had none of my own. My depression was a bottom. Relative to many others, it was a high bottom, but it was a bottom nonetheless. A bottom is often a wake up call as what we had been doing, by force of habit, no longer works. Reality is the leading cause of stress. Painful as it may be, we confront the actual reality of our situation. We become willing to change and may even enlist the services of others in support of that effort.

God as a Traveling Partner

Often, physicians have been so engaged by their patients who are willing to use their wake up call to heal their lives. Alone people may not feel capable of sustaining the effort required. A newfound willingness is born out of the ground of their acceptance. But, alone people may not feel capable of sustaining the effort required for the enterprise. "The enterprise is exploration into God" is a paradox. To explore God people need God. People need God as a traveling partner for the exploration into God. How do people do that? Albert Einstein is quoted as saying that when looking for an answer to a question the best answer is the simple one, not simpler. So, what does one do? God uses people. People, by virtue of their own willingness, to participate in loco parentis, in place of the parents, Father/Mother God.

Author Don Campbell once told a story about Jesus. It's about Jesus when he finished his work and returned home. God, the Father, said: "Son, I'm really proud of you. You did everything that I asked of you. And now you're back here with me. I'm delighted with what you accomplished and delighted to have you home. Now that you are back here with me, how will the plan go forward without you?" Jesus replied, "Well, as you know, I trained these disciples, about a dozen, to carry the work forward upon my return home. They are to carry the good news throughout the world." God commented, "That's great son. I appreciate the training that you did with those disciples. But, I was just wondering what contingency plan you put in place should that plan fail. What is plan B?" Jesus replied, "There is no plan B."

If there is no plan B, then people by virtue of their willingness self-select to participate in this healing work. It's not someone else's job. And people, just ordinary people, begin an exploration that penetrates through all manner of distractions, into the ultimate reality of God. Not some other worldly God above, but the Mystery that is present here and now, right in the middle of suffering. That connection cannot happen until people are willing to participate in Plan A and accept both the reality of what they need and what God needs.

People need God and ironically, God needs them. God needs them to be willing, to have a willingness to own their neediness so that they can be both receptacles to catch the healing waters and vessels for distribution.

Ways in which willingness might enhance your relationships with the chronically ill include:

- Start with yourself. Be open and willing to allow God to use you.
- Realize that if your patients are caretakers, they may find experiencing a chronic illness extremely difficult. Caretakers typically have trouble receiving care. Encourage caretaker patients to allow others to serve them. Explain to them that by doing so, others can participate in their life in a meaningful way. Ask the patient to at least take the first Step by asking a friend/relative to run an errand for them. It's a start on the road to emotional maturity.
- Take the time to explain to your patients that by being willing to ask others for help, they are calling forth the gifts of other people.
- Encourage patients to have a willingness to accept the illness as part of their lives. Stress that the illness doesn't define them as a person. Help them to recognize that they may be healing their lives through dealing with the process of their illness. The chronic illness has given them an excuse to see the familiar in new ways.

REFERENCES

1. John 5:1–6. *The New Oxford Annotated Bible*, Oxford University Press, 1991.
2. John 5:7. Ibid.

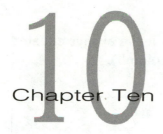

Chapter Ten

Principle 7: Humility

John A. Mac Dougall

> Walk not on the earth exultantly, for thou canst not cleave the earth, neither shalt thou reach to the mountains in height.
>
> The Koran, 17:37

Step Seven and the Humility Principle

Step Seven is: "Humbly asked Him to remove our shortcomings."

■ HUMILITY IS NOT ALWAYS POPULAR

It requires humility to be able to open up to change by a Higher Power. Humility is not popular, perhaps because it is often confused with humiliation. To achieve humility people must have an appropriate and realistic view of themselves, and be free of grandiosity and self-centeredness. Humility means that people realize that they are not God. People must recognize that they have no more right to all the good things of life than anyone else. All people are equal to every other human being and are loved and cared for by their Higher Power.

If people believe that they are better or more important than others, humility requires stepping down. This runs counter to values that they have been taught their whole lives. The world view may be built on competition and the belief that life is a zero sum game in which the gains of some people are always equaled by the losses of others (thus the name "zero sum").

■ THE WINNING CONCEPT

Growing up, I was taught that "Winning isn't the main thing, it's the only thing" and "Show me a good loser, and I'll show you a loser." I was in elementary school when the Soviet Union pulled ahead of America in the "Space Race" with the launch of the first satellite. We were told that our duty was to learn science so that America could catch up in space. Failure to win this race could result in nuclear annihilation. We studied and learned competition well. Fellowship works better than competition for spiritual growth. If we believe ourselves to be better than others, we will need to give up our grandiosity and special status in order to join the human race.

   If we believe we are worse than others, or less important, humility requires stepping up, in order to join the fellowship of the human race. Those who believe themselves to be less than others often pass up opportunities, on the theory that they are undeserving of the opportunities, or will be unsuccessful at them. Because of gender stereotypes, many men will have to step down to develop humility, and many women will have to step up.

■ THE "CIRCLE OF CONCERN"

There is a chart I call the "circle of concern." It is a circle, with a list of names. We are concerned about everyone inside the circle, and relatively unconcerned about everyone outside of it. Those who are grandiose have themselves inside of the circle, with everyone else outside of it unless they are consistently pleasing. Those who believe themselves unworthy have everyone else inside the circle, and themselves outside of it. A better view of this circle of concern is to have ourselves and all other people inside, with ourselves at the center and the people whom we love or for whom we have responsibility nearest to us. People we know less well take a more peripheral place, but are still inside the circle of concern. Humility comes with the belief that we are equal to every other human being: equal in status and equally within God's care. Sometimes, there are gender differences. Men more often need to include others in their circle of concern, and women more often need to include themselves, and not just the other people in their lives.

Time and Patience

Patience is an important tool in the development of humility. The grandiose person is rarely patient. Their motto is typically: "I want what I want when I want it. What I want is more, and when I want it is now." Their view of relationships can be expressed in the old nonsense: "When I say jump you jump, and ask how high on the way up!"

People need patience with time. This includes patience in traffic jams and supermarket lines. People can be patient with healing in their lives, and with spiritual growth itself. Patience is needed with other people. People are not God, and they don't have to obey other people's will. They don't have to take advice from others or direction, even if the others are "right." Instead of focusing on what other people should do to make their lives better, people should seek the help of a Higher Power for their own lives.

Asking for Help

The help from a Higher Power can be asked in the spirit of humility. The seventh Step of the Twelve Step programs is: "We humbly asked Him to remove our shortcomings." After willingness has been developed, it is time to ask for help.

This act of asking for help is an unusual type of prayer. The two most common types of prayer involve asking for things, and praying for other people. Children who pray often do both. These types of prayer come naturally. People tend to pray for things that they want, and that they have some difficulty getting all by themselves.

■ PRAYER REQUESTS

Because I have worked as a pastor, people have asked me to pray for favorable weather or for the victory of their sports team. I've joked and said I only do news, not sports or weather. I wasn't willing to advance the idea that God produces sunshine or sports scores on request.

People naturally pray for others, as an extension of their good will towards them. People don't pray for things they can handle themselves, but rather for things outside their control, like other people's health or safety. Children often are taught to pray for family members on a routine basis. What they don't tend to learn is to pray for their own spiritual growth and development.

The Seventh Step and Spiritual Growth

Having had the courage to examine their own consciences, the integrity to admit their wrongs, and the willingness to have their Higher Power change them, people take on a new prayer with humility. They pray that whatever is wrong be removed from their lives. People are praying for a change of heart, attitude, and behavior. The seventh step prayer of Alcoholics Anonymous (A.A.) has nothing to do with alcohol, and everything to do with spiritual growth. The experience of alcoholic men and women is that most have prayed to be sober, and gotten no results. As a result of praying for spiritual growth and change, sobriety followed. Their prayer reads: "My Creator, I am now willing that you should have all of me, good and bad. I pray that you now remove from me every single defect of character which stands in the way of my usefulness to you and my fellows. Grant me strength, as I go out from here, to do your bidding. Amen.''[1]

The Acceptance of Life Circumstances

This is a prayer of willingness and humility. In it, people pray not to have different things happen, or to get things, but to be different. It is intimidating because it is open ended. People ask to have their character defects removed without even being sure they have identified all of them. They ask without knowing how these character defects will be removed, and what the costs and consequences of change are.

Acceptance is a part of their willingness. People learn to accept themselves the way they are. People learn to live life on life's terms, not according to terms that they try to impose on it. This means that people must accept themselves regardless of physical and mental limitations, and must accept their emotions. People should accept others just the way they are, not the way they would be if they were perfectly designed. People must learn to accept life circumstances.

A Balanced, Centered Life Results from Humility

Acceptance doesn't mean approval. It simply means accepting the reality of things. Although people may still strive for improvement, acceptance means forgoing a sense of grievance and no longer acting as if people, places, and things were meant to obey their will.

Humility leads to lives that are balanced and centered. Humility leads to a way of life characterized by harmony and respect. The *Tao Te Ching* includes a poem about humility:

> The supreme good is like water,
> which nourishes all things without trying to.

It is content with the low places that people disdain,
Thus it is like the Tao.

In dwelling, live close to the ground.
In thinking, keep to the simple.
In conflict, be fair and generous.
In governing, don't try to control.
In work, do what you enjoy.
In family life, be completely present.

When you are content to be simply yourself
and don't compare or compete,
everybody will respect you.[2]

Being Real

The most important aspect of humility is the willingness for people to be who they actually are, today, at least as a starting point. They should be willing to accept their flaws, and to have their Higher Power remove them. People should be willing to accept the flaws in others, and not try to play God in their lives. Instead, others should be viewed and treated with compassion.

Suggestions for humility in your life and work:

- Humbly ask God to remove your shortcomings.
- View other people who work to help your patients as your equals, even if your skills exceed theirs.
- Encourage your patients to ask for help with both their spiritual concerns and physical concerns.
- Encourage your patients to see their illness as an opportunity to strip life of things that don't matter.
- Acknowledge the physical limitations that people have. Discourage patients from grading themselves on attractiveness, physical strength, resistance to disease, or speed of recovery.

Bowen F. White

There are many examples in recorded history of humility. Jesus is but one. But, even from a mythological perspective, his life is an impressive example of humility. In the Bible it says that God became a man in the person of Jesus. God became human. Now that's humility.

■ LIFE: A NEVER-ENDING LEARNING ENVIRONMENT

That example of humility may be difficult to relate to since it seems too far removed from people's database of life experience. When I hear someone like Gordon Cosby, a pastor of the Church of the Savior in Washington, D.C., speak, I think, "What the heck do I think I'm doing writing on this topic of spirituality? I'm not adequate to the task." That is how I feel. The part of me that has those feelings of inadequacy keeps reminding me that it is absurd to continue this writing because whatever I say, others could do it so much better. Many other people could write this book better than I. That's one reason that I asked John Mac Dougall to co-author this work. He is a clergy-man and very good at what he does at Hazelden. I am a medical doctor who has been naive enough to travel the spiritual path with suffering people. Why? Because they were there and we were both open to the value of the journey. An imperfect guide bumbling along with a sick person can sometimes be the right combination for new discoveries.

What I have seen has impressed me. In spite of my ineptness, rela-tive to others, patients have allowed me to watch as they faced their illness and taught me about humility. Early on, I thought my job was to teach them something. I was wrong. It took me a while but even-tually I realized that my real job is to create a safe learning environ-ment for gnosis. That way both of us gain some gnosis, some knowing, that neither of us had before. Or if we had it, we might have forgotten.

There is an old Sufi story that speaks to this forgetting. Sufism is an Islamic practice that centers on developing the abilities and hidden potential within each of us, so that we may come to live in harmony, unity, balance, love, and peace. A seeker is walking down the road and comes upon a rock. On the rock there is writing. The seeker looks down and reads, "turn me over to learn more." The seeker turns over the rock and reads, "why do you want to know more when you don't now use what you already know?" Why don't we use what we already know? I don't know about you, but I forget. I never forget to forget.

We've got to keep expanding the database and keep developing no matter what age we are. We never are finished learning and we never know it all. The more life experiences we have the more we discover how little we know and the more we develop. If people keep telling you how great you are, it's easy to forget that you don't know it all. It's important to keep our humility intact despite what others say to you.

I have a sign that I hung on my office door. It reads: "Caution. Beware of Doc. Enter at Your Own Risk. I Make Mistakes Every Day." I didn't put the sign on my office door for my patients. Instead, I put the sign on the office door for myself.

I did it because I make mistakes every day. And I want my patients to know, on the front end, that if they want a perfect doctor, I'm not the one to see. I don't think perfect is for human beings. I put the sign on the door nearly 15 years ago. Not one patient has seen the sign and walked out. The side effects with patients are priceless. They smile, relax, and trust is established almost instantaneously. By letting them know that I make mistakes every day, they feel more comfortable with me because they see me like themselves. I'm like them.

Connecting with Others

One of the problems clinicians have in the medical profession is that people may have difficulty connecting with them. Doctors are seen as different than regular people. Clinicians are the carriers of the secret knowledge taught during long arduous years of sacrifice at medical Meccas. Clinicians have a secret language that they acquired which demonstrates their learnedness. People often see clinicians from the perspective that they are at the top of the medical food chain and they are there for the crumbs. It's sad. In this litigious society clinicians can be even more paranoid about their own fallibility for want of safety from malpractice suits. The irony is that in letting patients know of their fallibility, if they feel that the clinicians sincerely care about them and are doing their best to serve, when they screw up, they don't go for the jugular. They understand that clinicians care and did what they could. People feel the clinician's caring. People don't want to be treated like numbers. They want to feel warmth coming from their caregiver. Malpractice suits occur most often when physicians and patients don't have good relationships.

This business of caring cannot be overstated. If people feel that they are being cared for, it changes everything. Despite what people are taught in medical school, it's OK to get emotionally involved. The less egocentric, the less clinicians let their ego drive their interactions, the more they can care for others. Instead of clinicians just caring about themselves they have energy to be used in the service of others.

A wonderful story that speaks about humility can be found in the May 10, 1999 issue of *Fortune* magazine. It is about Harry Pearce, the vice chairman of General Motors (GM), who has leukemia. The story "Can Leukemia Stop Harry Pearce from Running GM?" explained how this chronic illness affected his focus and subsequent energy flow. "You're less egocentric, because you realize in a very direct way how the support of others has contributed to your still being around. Your relationships with other people—your family, your friends, your fellow employees—become much more important," explained Harry. That doesn't mean that Harry didn't take care of himself. When his diagnosis was confirmed at Memorial Sloan-Kettering Cancer Center in NYC he was determined to do what he could to help himself. "That week I started an exercise program with treadmill and weights that was even more rigorous than the one I was on. My attitude was, I'm going to do everything known to man if it has even an incrementally positive impact. I walked every day, paid a lot of attention to what I ate, and gave up the occasional glass of wine since I learned that alcohol is a mild bone marrow depressant."

Humility doesn't preclude people taking care of themselves. It just helps them realize that the more broad their perspective is, the more healthy it is. Pearce explained, "When you get into an executive position, the tendency is to focus on your career. Not that I wasn't trying to do what was in the best interest of GM before, but it was too personalized. I don't have the same view today. I'm more likely now to make a decision based on the fundamental values."

Mr. Pearce fell off his metaphorical slack rope and got right back up with a renewed focus on the knot, "the fundamental values." It's not healthy for people to have one set of values for their work life and another set for their personal life. It's all one life. Sometimes people have to be brought to their knees, to be humbled, to remember humility and get back into alignment with their highest values. Pearce confessed, "I have never been one to wear religion on my sleeve, but you do a lot of soul-searching about what your beliefs really are. There is a strong bias to believe in God, because the alternative is a little bleak. It's something you can never logically resolve, but emotionally it provides tremendous support."

With humility, God is included in the equation. Although the rational mind cannot get its logic around the idea, "emotionally it provides tremendous support." Going on he says, "It gives you confidence that there's something out there working on your behalf beyond pure science. It causes you to focus on your own ethics and your own values more than you ever did."

The knot becomes the focal point of attention. It doesn't matter if it's at home or work. Attention and energy move in concert toward that which people hold to be most true. Work goes on, life goes on, but it goes on differently for the humble.

Poet William Blake said, "Pride is the cloak of knavery." There is a significant difference between being proud of the team, the group, and the organization versus being prideful, boastful. When Jesus said, "the meek shall inherit the earth" (Psalm 37:11) he wasn't talking about a death benefit. He was referring to a life benefit. Pastor Gordon at Church of the Savior referred to the kind of power that Jesus displayed as lamb power. It is a non-controlling kind of power. But, it is powerful nonetheless. The following poem by Rumi is about humility and lamb power. It describes this power concept well.

> You've seen a heard of goats going down to the river
> The lame and dreamy goat brings up the rear
> There are worried faces about that one
> But now they're laughing
> Because look, as they return
> that one is the leader
> There are many different ways of knowing
> The lame goats kind has branches that trace back to the roots
> of presence
> Learn from the lame goat
> and lead the herd home.

—Rumi

The lame, the sick, the chronically ill can demonstrate the kind of leadership that unites clinicians and patients with the best in all the healing traditions. Clinicians need to notice their own limping on the way to their ministrations. Who knows, perhaps people can be healed as they "learn from the lame goat and lead the herd home."

Ways in which you might incorporate humility in your life and in turn enhance your relationships with the chronically ill include:

- A bold step—put a sign on your office door like mine stating, "Caution. Beware of Doc. Enter at Your Own Risk. I Make Mistakes Every Day." Put the sign on the door not for your patients, but for yourself as a gentle reminder of your humanity.
- In your practice, start a mistake of the month meeting. We somehow forget that we learn from our mistakes. It's not enough to just honor our achievements.
- Recognize that freedom is not in being right. We can be self righteous because we are sure we are right. It is useful to remember that the truth doesn't need our defense. Hence, there is no need to be defensive.

- Take time to be with people that are at the margins of society—the poor and suffering. There are life lessons to be learned here. Encourage your patients to do the same.

REFERENCES

1. *Alcoholics Anonymous*, p. 76.
2. S. Mitchell, *Tao Te Ching, a New English Version*, Harper Collins, New York, 1992, p. 8.

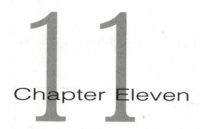

Chapter Eleven

Principle 8: Compassion

John A. Mac Dougall

> To be able to practice five things everywhere under heaven constitutes perfect virtue . . . gravity, generosity of soul, sincerity, earnestness, and kindness.
> *The Confucian Analects*, book 17:6

> What is hateful to you do not do to your neighbor. That is the whole Torah. The rest is commentary.
> Hillel, 30 B.C.– A.D. 10

Step Eight and the Compassion Principle

Step Eight states: "Made a list of all persons we had harmed, and became willing to make amends to them all."

Avoiding Self-Centeredness

Spiritual progress so far can be seen as a movement away from natural self-centeredness. Self-centeredness is natural because people perceive the world from inside of themselves. People look through their own eyes, feel their own pain, and make their own plans. They automatically love what they love and it is only with effort that they learn to love what others love. It is only natural to believe that others are either just like them or defective. It is only with experience and practice that they can begin to see things from other people's point of view.

■ THE MIRROR AND THE COFFEEMAKER

The first Christmas after I was married to my wife, Priscilla, I bought her a good automatic coffeemaker for Christmas. I was sure she'd like it because it used the paper filters that removed bitterness from coffee. She got me a full length mirror because I didn't have one, and could not fully appreciate how I looked in the morning. We received each others' gifts with a distinct lack of joy. I rapidly discovered that she doesn't drink coffee. She in turn discovered that I don't care how I look in the morning. If I have clothes on I consider the task of getting dressed accomplished.

It Matters

The prerequisite to having compassion for others is the humility to believe that other people's wants, needs, and perceptions matter. As long as a person believes that they are the center of the universe, the meaning of compassion naturally becomes that other people ought to have compassion for them. As they mature, they discover an interest in their fellow human beings, and a desire to see how their actions affect them. Some of this is influenced by gender roles and stereotypes. Men may need to learn that other people's wants, needs, and perceptions matter. Women may need to learn that their own wants, needs, and perceptions matter, and they may benefit from developing some compassion for themselves.

Compassion has to do with a person's ability to suffer with others. First they have to believe that other people matter. Then they need to consider life from other people's point of view. Once they understand other people's pain and distress, they may discover that they have played a part in creating or sustaining it. Humility teaches people that they are the equal of other people. Compassion teaches people that the force that unites them is mutual affection and support.

Restoring Damaged Relationships ....

Spirituality has to do with the quality and nature of people's relationships in three dimensions: with a Higher Power, themselves, and with others. This continues the restoration of their damaged relationships.

This resembles the examination of conscience completed while developing courage in Chapter 7. However, the focus is somewhat different. People had the courage to assess what they had done wrong. Now they need the compassion to assess the effects they have had on others. This is not necessarily related to what they have done wrong. They may have been arguably right and still have harmed people. They need to consider the impact they have had on others independent of the moral nature of their actions. Instead of simply evaluating their conduct, they look at how their being and doing impacts others.

Learning how others feel prepares people to make peace with others and live in harmony. Then, they are able to move beyond judgment of their guilt or innocence, and accept responsibility for any harm they have done, regardless of the reason they have done it. For the purposes of this phase of spiritual development, intentions matter little. The bottom line is whether they have harmed people or not despite the intention.

If someone is hit by a bus while crossing the street and their hip is broken as a result, the accident has impacted them although it wasn't their fault. If someone is hit by a drunk driver and their hip is broken as a result, the impact is very similar, even though the blame is shifted. If they are attacked by someone with a baseball bat and their hip is broken, the physical impact is the same. However, they may be more upset than the other injured people because the injury was intentional, but there are major aspects of the harm that are the same, regardless of intent.

As people develop compassion for others, they ask how they have harmed people on purpose. They may have been operating out of self-centeredness, and put people down in the hopes of improving their own lives. They may have gossiped about and criticized others. They may have treated others as actors in a play of their authorship, having meaning only as they carry out the roles they have assigned for others.

■ THE POWER OF GRIEF LETTERS

In 1989, I was involved in a grief group. Here a man wrote a grief letter to a young man he had killed during the Nazi invasion of Poland. The man writing the grief letter had been a resistance fighter armed with a hunting rifle during the war. One day as the man walked alone over the hill he encountered a single German soldier who appeared to be just a teenager. Both aimed and fired at each other and the man killed the young German soldier. The man wrote in his grief letter that he had killed many more men in the course of the war, but this first one always stuck out in his mind. He wrote of the grief of taking another man's life and the sorrow it must have brought to a German family. He cried, as did all who listened. He had put this young German soldier on his list of those he had harmed. In turn he developed compassion for the soldier and his family. It was good.

■ OPENING UP

As I continue my development, I ask how I have harmed others by mistake. As an ambulance driver, I was once called to a car wreck where two men were badly hurt. I crawled through the broken back window and got behind the driver. Because the door was crushed, he couldn't be removed until the passenger was taken out. I monitored his vital signs while the other medics splinted the passenger. As the driver began to fail, I ordered the other medics to remove the passenger even though he hadn't been properly splinted and wasn't ready to be moved. The results of that decision were poor. The driver died anyhow in the hospital and the passenger's injuries were made much worse by moving him prematurely.

One could argue that I wasn't wrong and that my intentions were good. That's true, but I still harmed the passenger. A sense of self-justification would have hardened my heart against feeling his pain. The truth was that his pain was increased and his sadness compounded by the death of his friend. Visiting him in the hospital and allowing myself to be sad with him kept me open to life.

Harming Others Through Omission

The next step is for people to ask how they have harmed others by omission. Here again, they may not be morally wrong, but their lack of action or compassion has caused others harm. Alan D., who was abused as a child, took pride in the fact that he never abused his own children. He had broken the cycle of abuse. However, when his children grew into teens he realized that he had omitted many opportunities for tenderness and kindness. While focusing on doing what he shouldn't do, he had missed opportunities for love and friendship along the way.

Letting Go of Excuses and Blame

Being a victim is irrelevant to the need to develop compassion and the need to list those people who have been harmed. Spiritual growth is not advanced by excuses or blame. Sometimes when Alan D. would try to tell others about his childhood abuse, the listeners would immediately assume that Alan's abusers must have had bad childhoods themselves. Alan then would state that he didn't care. After all, these people were all responsible for their actions, regardless of what has happened to them in the past. His childhood abuse wasn't an excuse for the harm he had done and other people's possible abuse wasn't an excuse for their harm. Letting go of excuses and blame allows each person to grow spiritually.

The Gift of Forgiveness

There is a role for forgiveness in the development of compassion. Forgiveness isn't a duty, it is a gift. It is difficult to choose to forgive others and then make it come true. Forgiveness is more the activity of a gracious Higher Power allowing them to release resentments. Forgiveness is sometimes objectionable because it can have the implication that the offense is somehow acceptable. A common attempt at forgiveness is sometimes phrased as "Oh, that's all right."

Forgiveness is most valuable when applied to things that are not "all right" at all. Forgiveness is releasing an attachment to resentment, hatred, and revenge. A popular slogan is "Forgiveness is giving up hope for a better past." Without forgiveness, people are likely to be too full of anger to have room to understand and identify with the feelings of others. With it, they may discover compassion even for those who have harmed them. In a letter about his abuse, Alan D. wrote: "Just as it was sad to be a little boy who was beaten, it must have been sad to be a mother who beats her little boy." People do not need to like or accept people in order to have compassion. Instead, they need to ask their Higher Power for the ability to have forgiveness and compassion, not for the other person's sake, but for their own.

Having Compassion for Themselves

As a person makes a list of all the people they've harmed, they need to include themselves on the list. In the case of chronic illness, they may have harmed themselves along the way: participating in the onset of the illness through their behaviors, neglecting treatment, or condemning themselves for being ill. People with illnesses that are consequences of addiction need to have compassion on themselves rather than harshly judging themselves for failing to quit alcohol, nicotine, or other drugs. Out of that compassion, they may grant themselves treatment opportunities for the addiction and for the secondary diseases that flow from addictions. Failing to have compassion, they may misunderstand the natural consequences of the disease process, believing the harm to be their just punishment. People with advanced illnesses that could possibly have been treated much earlier can have compassion on themselves and seek treatment in the present rather than "kicking themselves" for not starting sooner.

A good treatment for shame and guilt is for a person to develop compassion for themselves and others. People often treat the shame of being uncaring by becoming caring. Others prepare to treat the guilt of causing harm by becoming willing to make amends.

Again, the spiritual principle of willingness is crucial. People need to become willing to make amends to all the people they have harmed. Often, they may not be willing. Instead, they may be looking for a chance to harm others again.

■ BECOMING HARMLESS

Even such a small scale enterprise as office gossip has an important element of harm in it. A friend of mine who is a medical school professor jokes that the reason academic politics are so vicious is because the stakes are so small. When we aren't spiritually fit, no stakes are too small for us to fight over. As we develop compassion, we begin to change and we become harmless people.

Reassessing Life

People reassess life with a sense of compassion for themselves and others. They apply the spiritual principles of anonymity and humility, and learn to give every single human being a high value. With compassion, they know what people need, and what needs are going unmet. Out of compassion, they begin to want justice, healing, and the restoration of relationships for themselves and others.

Suggestions for compassion in your life and work:

- Eat and sleep. Compassion fatigue is linked to physical fatigue. You cannot effectively promote other people's health by ruining your own.
- Make a list of all persons you have harmed, and become willing to make amends to them all.
- Encourage your patients to have compassion for health care providers, family members, and other caregivers. Inform them that hostile or divisive behavior on their part makes them spiritually and physically sick.
- Encourage your patients to have compassion for themselves. Symptoms of their diseases are not judgments on them. Hospitalized patients do not have to be responsible for hospitality to all visitors at all hours.
- Reduce the practice of defensive medicine. Use your mistakes as learning occasions for yourself and teaching moments for your colleagues.

Bowen F. White

A side effect of having cancer was that GM Vice Chairman, Harry Pearce became more compassionate. "I've become a much stronger advocate of teamwork, and I have more compassion for others. Whereas, in the past you would have gotten frustrated with somebody when you were trying to explain something to them and they didn't get it—that wouldn't happen now." His illness changed him and compassion grew as a result. "There has been a very real transformation in how I think. Even people I didn't care for in the past, I find myself reexamining and looking for the good, and often finding it. This experience focuses your attention on what I call real value."

Here's Harry, chasing the American dream and grasping it at the highest level of achievement and recognition vis-à-vis the world of business. He was on the verge of a promotion and then his world stopped. The flashlight of his attention moved. "This experience focuses your attention on what I call real value." And he looks anew at people in his life to include those he did not like. He looks for the good, the value in others and often finds what he is looking for.

■ MORE THAN FACING DEATH, GETTING RELIGION

I shared the material on GM's Harry Pearce with a leadership group at a division of a Fortune 500 company. One of the participants was not impressed with Harry Pearce's story. His comment was something like, "Big deal. It's just another story of someone facing death and getting religion. If he weren't a big deal at GM there'd be no story. I'd be more impressed if someone changed without such drama." Another participant seconded his comments.

It is interesting that what some in this audience wanted was a story that would move them. This one didn't do that. Maybe that's what we all want. The story that will move us to be the person we are capable of being. Frankly, I don't believe it's another story that they, and we, want at all. We want to keep doing what we have been doing and find reasons to poke holes in any story that might suggest we change. We rationalize being stuck.

Living Life to the Fullest

What seems to be required is a story that includes people in a very personal way. Do people have to look death in the face to live life to the fullest? No, but something has to touch them where they live to get their attention. Maybe using author Stephen Mitchel's definition of compassion will help. Mitchel said that when love touches suffering the result is compassion. Whereas, when people's fear touches suffering pity results.

Love is the key word. What fullness can life have without love?

■ WHEN LOVE ENTERS

Think of your own life. Think of the changes in your own life that happened when love entered. And now think of how you felt when love departed. Love enters and we feel capable of anything. Love is lost and we are lost. Love returns and we are inspired, full of creative energy. Love leaves and we cannot imagine a creative act.

So it is not just in facing death that we wake up to living life fully. But, also in loving that fullness is experienced. So, there are similarities. There are also differences as well. We face death alone. Love, on the other hand, is a shared experience. We die alone. We love together. Attending the dying with love allows both the living and dying to feel the loving energy. But, the dying person experiences death while feeling loved. The attending loving person feels compassion for the dying while loving them. Each is focused. Each is changed. It is a sacred moment, a full moment for each. Knotted together by compassion both suffer love fully.

Patients Need Compassion, Not Pity

Clinicians have probably seen some of their patients respond like Harry while others have not experienced this kind of "transformation." Clinicians may not know how other patients responded because they didn't spend the time necessary to explore the meaning of the illness with the patient. Regardless, all patients in the clinician's care need compassion, not pity.

If it is the clinician's fear that touches their suffering, they sense pity and may feel pitiful. That is unempowering. Patients will feel safe with their clinicians when the clinicians exude a loving warmth that comforts and empowers. Love power/lamb power is the ultimate source of safety. As clinicians surrender personal power by giving up having to have things work out their way, clinicians in turn release fear that has been the driver of their behavior. It is their fear that has no faith in the unfolding of the future. When they release fear, love rushes into the vacuum. Brimming with a new fullness, compassion replaces pity as love embraces the suffering patient.

■ AN ENCOUNTER WITH THE DALAI LAMA

In 1989, I went to a medical meeting in Bangalore, India. The first speaker at that meeting was the Dalai Lama, leader of the Tibetan people. I had a press pass from my local newspaper to do an interview with His Holiness, as he is called. I wanted some special time alone with him and figured the press credential would give me some leverage to gain same.

I sat on the front row as the Dalai Lama began his presentation. He started out by saying that he had no idea why he was speaking at a medical meeting. He talked about one thing that he had learned in his 30 years as a refugee, you cannot pretend things are different than they are. The actual reality is that he didn't know anything about medicine. He said that sometimes he gets sick and goes to see the doctor. It may be a top specialist with many degrees on the wall. But, if he doesn't feel any warmth coming from the doctor, it doesn't matter. He doesn't feel so good. On the other hand, if he gets sick and goes to see the doctor, just a regular doc and he feels warmth, it doesn't really matter what medicine the doctor gives him, he feels better. In retrospect, I think he knew a great deal about medicine! At the conclusion of his lecture, he talked about the current world situation. Although I saw the lecture about ten years ago, it still pertains today. He said that if one looks at the world it is clear that what is required is love and compassion. Religion is a luxury. Regardless of the era, what is required in the world is love and compassion. You probably won't find that in your job description as a clinician. If you get sick, do you want cold or warmth coming your direction? Gandhi said to be the dream you want to see in the world. Arise from your slumber and dream your life. And the knot will be clearly in focus.

I never did ask for the private interview with the Dalai Lama. Hearing him speak to our group for 30 minutes was enough. I felt as if I had been to the well and was full already.

Ways in which you might use compassion in your everyday life which will in turn enhance your relationships with the chronically ill include:

- Embrace your patients in an unconditional, positive regard.
- Create an environment where the patient feels safe. Attempt to make them feel less alone and less frightened by treating each and every patient with love and compassion.
- Suggest that your chronically ill patients interact with others in a similar situation by joining a support group.
- Recognize there is a difference between pity and compassion. Suffering and love equals compassion, but suffering and fear equal pity.
- Really look at how you treat people in everyday life. First, look at yourself. Remember to love thy neighbor as thyself.
- Quit being so cruel to yourself despite all your flaws and mistakes. Live in a love based relationship instead of a fear based relationship.

- Love by definition is non-controlling. If you act in a controlling manner, it's not love. You have control over whether or not you feel love. There is something healing about loving. The more people you love, the better you feel.

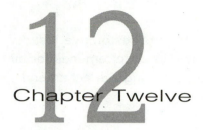

Chapter Twelve

Principle 9: Justice

John A. Mac Dougall

Do justice, that you may live long upon the earth. Calm the weeper, do not oppress the widow, do not oust a man from his father's property, do not degrade magnates from their seats. Beware of punishing wrongfully; do not kill, for it will not profit you.

The Teaching for Merikare, par. 8, c. 2135–2140 B.C.

Step Nine and the Justice Principle

Step Nine states: "Made amends to such people wherever possible, except when to do so would injure them or others."

What Justice Means to Spiritual Growth

Once people have compassion for others, and can see how they have harmed them, it is time for justice. When they think of justice, they often think of criminal law and the detection of crime, the apprehension of suspects, the determination of guilt or innocence according to law, and the punishment of the guilty. Another model is civil law, in which losses are reimbursed and equity restored. For the purposes of spiritual growth, people need to go beyond civil and criminal law to restorative justice. The elements of restorative justice include direct amends for all people who have been harmed by them, making indirect amends, and gift-giving.

Chronic Illness as a Punishment

Sometimes people take the analogy of criminal law and apply it to chronic illness. They mistake the symptoms of their disease for punishment for their wrongdoings. This is often based on a traditional religious view that good behavior results in good health. In the New Testament, the words for salvation and health are the same. The belief was that illness was the result of sin and that getting right with God would cure illness. People with a chronic illness will often ask, "Why me? I've been good." or "What have I done to deserve this?" It is important to tell them that illness and wrongdoing are different. People who have done a lot of drugs will take their symptoms and attribute them to the wrongdoing of drug taking rather than to the disease of chemical dependency. An alcoholic with cirrhosis of the liver may see it as God's punishment for drinking. He may continue drinking to treat the pain of being punished by God instead of getting sober and letting the liver heal. Some women who have had abortions fear that God will punish this perceived wrongdoing with a later inability to have children. Then, if they fail to become pregnant when they want to, they quietly hide their shame and God's perceived punishment instead of seeking infertility treatment. A heart attack patient may perceive chest pains as punishment for a bad lifestyle instead of getting treated and taking action to prevent further problems.

Chronic Illness as Compensation

Using civil law as an analogy for illness represents slight progress. Instead of seeing symptoms as punishment, people may see them as just compensation for unhealthy lifestyle choices. Even this model leads to a sense of defeat. Consequences can be seen as justice rather than symptoms of disease and guides to treatment.

Restorative justice is a good analogy for illness. People cooperate in the diagnosis of what's wrong and then take action to either treat and cure it, or adapt to its presence in their lives. People make direct amends with direct treatment, indirect amends with successful adaptation to chronic illness and resumption of healthy lifestyles, and give gifts to themselves in the wake of the opportunities that illness provides for the reevaluation of life.

Restorative Justice is Good for Spirituality and Resilience

The Twelve Step Programs realize that restorative justice is good for spirituality and resilience. The Ninth Step reads: "We made direct amends to such people wherever possible, except when to do so would injure them or others." Having made a list of all persons they have harmed, including themselves, they set out to restore justice to their lives.

Making Amends

To be spiritually well, people make direct amends to the people they have harmed on purpose. Out of their own defects of character, they have hurt people. If they think back to the defects of character that they identified with courage and admitted to with integrity, they will know how to make amends. For example, if they have been angry and lashed out with words or actions, they apologize and accept responsibility for their actions. They do not attribute any aspect of their angry outbursts to the other person, even if they could justify it to themselves by saying "they made me angry." They have been angry at others, but the responsibility for their actions is theirs, nobody elses.

Making Direct Amends

If there is material harm, people try to make direct amends and restore it. If they have stolen from or defrauded anyone, they pay them back. If they have done injury, they offer to pay for the treatment of that injury, whether physical or emotional. This could include doctor bills or therapy. Direct amends involve paying them directly, with an acknowledgment that they are doing it in order to bring justice back to the relationship.

They make direct amends to the people they have harmed by accident. If they have been insecure in the past, and out of that insecurity engaged in a pattern of gossip and criticism, they apologize and admit to the dynamics of insecurity and criticism. They go beyond stating that they are sorry, and tell the persons they have harmed exactly why they have done it. This is not an excuse, but rather evidence that they understand what they have done and are ready to stop. They may not have set out to harm others, but in the process of bolstering their own egos they may have harmed others nonetheless.

When people do physical harm to others in an accident, they have insurance to provide financial amends. They may not have committed any moral wrongdoing, but through an accident they have done harm, and taking responsibility is good for them. Many insurance policies provide for payment for injuries to others, regardless of fault. People then can take responsibility for the harm caused, even if they didn't intend to cause it.

People Harmed by Omission

People working Principle 9 make direct amends to those they have harmed by omission. These are people that have been harmed without the person even thinking about it. Other people might have needed help and the person wasn't available to see it or simply forgot about it. They could say they were not at fault because they forgot, but the harm is real to the other person nonetheless. Married couples often omit romance and overt expressions of love on the theory that the other person "ought to know" they love them. Leaving specific expressions of love out of relationships creates as much harm as anger or rejection.

Admitting Harm to Themselves and Others

In addition to making direct amends to others, people make amends to themselves for the ways in which they have harmed themselves. It is difficult to admit that they sometimes harm themselves on purpose. When depressed, people use the answering machine to screen their calls knowing that they are making their depression and isolation worse, but they do it anyway. When suicidal, they are planning or carrying out harm against themselves. When very angry, they sometimes injure themselves as "stand-ins" for the people they would really like to injure. Amends would involve answering the phone, reestablishing healthy relationships, and living well instead of being self-destructive.

Learning to Respect Themselves

It is more common to harm themselves by mistake. Denial of risk can keep harms from being "on purpose," but they are harmful, just the same. If they have had a bad diet, no exercise, lots of cigarettes, and chest pain, they might change their lifestyle in a way that would promote recovery. If they have been drinking and drugging, they don't just quit, instead they actively pursue a Twelve Step program in order to become clean and sober, not just abstinent. If people have been compulsively overspending, they develop a plan for paying their credit card balances and take the action to open retirement accounts on the grounds that there actually is a tomorrow following today. People also harm themselves by omission. They may have avoided appropriate risks at work or in relationships out of an ineffective attempt to shield themselves from pain. While shielding themselves from the pain, they also managed to shield themselves from opportunity. They make amends by stepping out and asserting themselves to reach their goals.

The Exception

The exception to direct amends is when the process of amends would cause fresh injury, either to themselves or to others. In the case of having an extramarital affair, amends would not include running home to confess to their partner because that would injure the innocent party. Indirect amends would involve quietly ending the affair, and also bringing one's energy, love, and commitment back home. This involves ending the harm, restoring the estrangement, and changing into the kind of person who keeps commitments. Rekindling the betrayed relationship and rediscovering what led them to make a commitment in the first place is a good start.

Another example is if a person has been secretly critical of others and they are unaware of the harshness, they don't reveal it to the others because that would harm them. Hurting another person to feel better is wrong. Along the same lines, hurting themselves in the pursuit of justice is useless. Overweight people who try to make amends through crash dieting harm themselves. The profligate who becomes stingy is doing no one a favor. The goal of amends is balance and justice, not punishment.

Restoring Balance Through Indirect Amends............................

If direct amends are inappropriate because of the harm they would cause, then indirect amends could be in order. In many cases, the indirect amends are more important than the direct ones. As mentioned previously in Chapter 2 on spirituality, indirect amends consist of someone first changing their behavior on that issue, and ultimately involve changing their character with the help of peers, programs, and a Higher Power.

Through direct amends others are reimbursed for what has been taken from them. People apologize for what they have done wrong and attempt to restore balance to the relationship. Changes are made to their actions. An attempt to restore balance also occurs with indirect amends, but because of the circumstances, they are done so in an indirect or symbolic way. It is done this way in order to avoid harming anyone. Ultimately, the most important amends are to change who they are, with the help of their Higher Power and friends.

■ AN ADDITIONAL FIFTH STEP

An example of indirect amends to others came from a man who returned to Hazelden for an additional Fifth Step. He met with me after stating it would only be a short visit. He just had one thing to say, which he left out of his original Fifth Step, and it had been bothering him. This secret was making it difficult for him to recover. He then confessed that he had embezzled $20,000 from his employer. He hadn't wanted to talk about it because he was afraid of making direct amends. A confession might result in prosecution and imprisonment, and then there would be no one to support his family.

I stated that the Fifth Step was just about admitting his wrongs, not about doing something about them. Integrity could be achieved by telling me the truth. He experienced a sense of relief. I then suggested we look ahead at possible amends. I agreed with him that direct amends would injure others in this case. I then went on to inquire about indirect amends. I asked, "Who was really harmed here? Who would have gotten the benefit of the money stolen?" It turns out that the money came from a fund intended for corporate charity. In truth, it would have benefited people in need, not the company itself. An embezzlement loss was as tax deductible as a charitable contribution, so ultimately there was no harm to the company. Instead, the harm was to the people who would have benefited from the charity.

The man was currently in a position to pay back the $20,000. I suggested that he purchase $20,000 worth of treatment for chemical dependency from another treatment facility, near the business in question, and then offer the "gift certificates" to the judge of the district court where he lived to be used for the benefit of people in court who needed to go to treatment but didn't have the money. By making this anonymous gift he would pay back what he had stolen in a way that would bring benefit to the public and honor his own recovery. He was happy with the suggestion and later wrote to tell me he had completed the task and was experiencing excellent sobriety as a result. He brought justice, balance, and restoration to his life and the lives of others through making indirect amends.

The Gift of Happiness

When people make indirect amends it leads to giving gifts to both themselves and others. Instead of stopping when they're "even," they go beyond justice to graciousness. They give, not just to compensate for wrongs, but because giving increases happiness all around. It was just for the man to give the $20,000 he embezzled in a way that benefited others. It also gave him insight into the happiness of giving and he continued to support causes that benefited others and made him feel happy. Generosity is good treatment for theft.

■ APOLOGIZING FOR UNREASONABLE CRITICISMS

I had a parishoner who had severe arthritis. She was older and living with her adult daughter and grandchildren. Years ago, she began to displace her anger at her pain and limited mobility onto her family. She constantly criticized them for how they lived. She denounced her daughter's parenting, her grandchildren's exuberant behavior, and the entire family for not caring about her. I was able to meet with her and clarify that it was her own physical distress that she hated, not her family. She called a family meeting and made amends, accepting responsibility for her unreasonable criticisms. She asked her family to help her avoid dumping on them by asking her what's wrong when she became hostile in the future. Gradually, she was able to extinguish most of her complaining. In turn, her relationships at home became more loving. She also reported that she had less pain. Her assessment was that by dwelling on the pain she had made it worse. She said, "I still don't like being old and sick, but I'm grateful to have my family."

The Gifts of Recovery

It is useful for the addict and alcoholic to stop drinking and drugging. But getting clean and sober is only a beginning of all the gifts that can come in recovery. By continuing in a program of spiritual growth, life can be better than it would have been if they had never been addicted.

■ LEARNING TO VALUE LIFE

If someone told me that there was a pill I could take that would treat my addiction, I would lack interest. If they said that with this new medication, I could be a social drinker, do a few recreational drugs now and then, and wouldn't need meetings, I wouldn't want it. I value the spiritual way of life I have learned and would not go back to "normal," even if I could. I don't work Twelve Step programs just to treat my diseases, but choose the programs as a way of life that is more satisfying than normal.

What Is Really Important in Life

It is useful for the coronary artery disease patient to get effective treatment and make lifestyle changes. By continuing in a program of spiritual growth, patients can make a virtue out of adversity, and use the brush with death as a reason for renewing life.

As patients, it is good to treat a disease and arrest or reverse it, but an additional opportunity is provided. The "time out" of illness allows an evaluation of what's really important in life. People can give the gift of thoughtful use of time, both to themselves and others. They begin to treat life as precious after the life threatening event.

In theory, people could grow spiritually and give good gifts to themselves and others without the challenges of chronic illness, but personal growth seems to come better from adversity than from ease. Adversity teaches perseverance, and if people will persevere in their development, life will continue to get better.

Suggestions for justice in your life and work:

- Make direct amends to the people you have harmed, unless to do so would injure them or others.
- Be just in your treatment of employees and colleagues.
- Do what you reasonably can to bring justice in the face of an inequitable health care system.
- Encourage your patients to look for ways in which they have been unjust, and to make their own amends. This helps them prepare to both die and live well.
- Interpret your patients' illness as diseases, rather than as cosmic justice or injustice.

Bowen F. White

"In other words, God 'justifies' (read 'validates') creation not by parental punishment from without, but by positive enticement and transformation from within. Surely a far greater victory and achievement of 'justice' on God's part. This concept of grace is first called mercy, HESED, the ever faithful, covenant-bound love of God. I would go so far as to call it THE PRIMARY REVELATION of the Bible."[1]

This view of justice will be explored here. As a spiritual principle it is core knot material. Or, as Rohr states, it is "the primary revelation of the Bible." And it is the result of the merciful grace of God. The light and dark in people is projected out to others. No one is all light or all dark. People have to accept this about everyone they meet, marry, doctor, lead, serve, parent, manage, report to, befriend, befoe, mentor, ask to mentor us, hire, fire, or otherwise interact with. People do not have to accept this about everyone but it might be healthier for all if they did.

People are made in the image of God. There is no Great Psychologist, Great Social Worker, or Great Clinician. Humans are not all light. They have their radiance, their light aspect, just as the moon reflects the light of the sun. But, people also have the shadow, analogous to the dark side of the moon. But people have trouble integrating both aspects into a whole, healthy, emotionally mature human being. The light people see in another person, the radiance of another, cannot be seen if it weren't also in that person. At times the wonderfulness that people see in others is just another reason to feel bad about themselves. People compare themselves to others and feel inadequate. They may feel that others are radiant and they, by comparison, are dull.

The irony is, once again, an illness or other status-quo-breaking life experience may help them move in the direction of real health. This means that someone can get sick and be healthier than someone else walking down the street without any known disease. Was it fair that Harry Pearce got sick? Was it just? He had a right to complain. But, he chose not to and instead chose to see the world differently than before the illness.

As in the sun and moon analogy, humans are like the moon in relation to the sun, God. Their shadow side contains those negative aspects of themselves that they have not accepted as theirs. Without self-acceptance they cannot integrate these elements into their awareness. They cannot shine the flashlight of their attention on something they are perceptually unaware of as theirs and then do something about it. Instead they shine the flashlight outside themselves. People see the character flaws of other people and vow never to be like them. In reality, that exact character flaw may be present in their own shadow too. They then project their shadow onto others and darken them. Often, they think that others are the problem in their life. They want others to change. They think that then everything will be better.

For example, if someone states, "I can't stand greedy people." Having named the flaw, they can then claim it. This means that if they are honest with themselves, they have to admit that at times they are greedy too. They don't want to see themselves as greedy because that is an unacceptable trait for them. However, they realize that at times they are greedy and so they claim the flaw.

By owning the flaw people can with honest humility see the others as similar, not different. They are like them. The flaw connects them with an opportunity to learn something about themselves. And accepting that they have the ability to be greedy, they can watch with an enlightened eye their own behavior. And keeping the observer eye focused on their own behavior, they have provided energy to keep their greediness from being acted out.

Somewhere along the line in human cultural evolution people's highest spiritual values have to become inculcated into all aspects of living. People cannot wait for politicians to lead the way on this. Nor can they wait for any other group to get with the health agenda instead of the death agenda. Clinicians should inform their patients that even spiritual healers can be suspect. Recently, a so-called "spiritual healer" described his work with a cancer patient, a woman with breast cancer. He said that surgery had been recommended by her doctor, but he, the healer, was advising against such a procedure. He went on to say that her problem, as with all women with breast cancer, was that she had not been nurturing enough to herself. She had always been the caregiver and had been neglectful of her needs throughout her life. He concluded that she didn't need surgery. Instead, she needed to start to nurture herself. By stating that her cancer was her fault and she could have avoided it by taking better care of herself, she became doubly damaged—once by the cancer and again by the spiritual healer. By making her feel guilty for her cancer she had yet another reason to feel bad. If she followed his advice and the illness ran its course downhill, then each step would become another failure on her part. She will begin to think that if she only nurtured herself better, if she had only had more faith, if she were only somehow different than she was, then she would have been able to beat that cancer.

He was not doing his client justice. And if she has a resectable tumor, his advice could hasten her death. That is a disservice. That is malpractice. Clinicians cannot assume that it is someone else's job to discuss spiritual matters with those that they serve. Clinicians may think that they are not up to the task. Maybe they aren't up to embarking on a spiritual journey with their patient. Realize that maybe there is no one else for the patient to turn to. The clinician should at least make the inquiry on whether the patient is receiving spiritual support. Even self-proclaimed spiritual healers may not be as useful as a blundering clinician that is open to being a tool of service.

This particular spiritual healer used a simplistic approach with his breast cancer client. His set of biases was the all or none set. The spiritual healer truly believed that all women with breast cancer got it because they were always nursing, caring for others while neglectful of themselves. Clinicians, at least in medicine, have learned that they never say "never" and they never say "always." The breast cancer patient may need to learn to nurture herself. But, that doesn't mean she doesn't also need to have surgery.

People have to see what soothes, what heals, what comforts them and thereby gain the insight to determine how to justly treat others. A very old prayer that has served this function is the Jesus prayer: "Lord Jesus Christ have mercy on me." Great numbers of seekers have found this simple prayer to be just what they need to remember what is important for the just treatment of both self and others—mercy. The prayer is only seven words. If people are uncomfortable with the words "Jesus Christ," they may substitute them with "God Almighty." This prayer is a simple way of staying focused on the knot.

Clinicians can be instruments of mercy as they use their gifts in the service of suffering people. For some of them, those gifts include the manual dexterity of the skilled surgeon. Why deny the expression of those gifts that can be so useful in the just treatment of another in a mission of mercy?

How the principle of justice may enhance all your relationships, including those chronically ill patients under your care might include:

- Start by not judging your patients. Instead, look at forgiveness and redemption. Ask your patients to look at who they need to forgive. Explain that everyone needs mercy and they don't need to earn it. Everyone should be allowed to live a graceful life and be given the benefit of the doubt.
- We can be instruments of healing. Something healing for us happens when we decide not to be judging. When we are judgmental, we make others feel uncomfortable.
- Don't discriminate who should get what. It's not your job to judge. Be merciful and full of mercy.

REFERENCE

1. Richard Rohr, *Job and the Mystery of Suffering: Spiritual Reflections*, Crossroad Pub. Co., 1997, p. 57.

13

Chapter Thirteen

Principle 10: Perseverance

John A. Mac Dougall

> Failure is an opportunity.
> If you blame someone else,
> there is no end to the blame.
>
> Therefore the Master
> fulfills her own obligations
> and corrects her own mistakes.
> She does what she needs to do
> and demands nothing of others.
>
> *Tao Te Ching*[1]

Step Ten and the Perseverance Principle

The Tenth Step is: "Continued to take personal inventory and when we were wrong promptly admitted it."

Letting Go of the Past

If people have been thorough with these spiritual principles, life should be reasonably satisfying. No longer do they live with "emotional hangovers." These hangovers take place when current, unpleasant emotions are based in past events. When people live in a state of reaction against people, places, and things they expend about 40 percent of our energy in the past, in the form of resentment and regret. Another 40 percent of their energy is expended into the future in the form of anxiety and worry. They end up living with only about 20 percent of their energy in the present. As their spiritual life improves, and their attitude and outlook on life change, they live with about 5 percent of their energy in the past, in the form of respect for their heritage. They put 5 percent of their energy in the future, in the form of planning. They then have about 90 percent of their energy available for living in the moment.

People in Twelve Step programs become honest and have hope, faith, and courage. They have developed the integrity to take responsibility for themselves, and the willingness to be changed for the better. They have the humility to live in fellowship with the rest of the human race, and they have compassion for their fellows. They have become just and this is a good way of life.

They have discovered that living according to spiritual principles will address all their problems. They will solve some problems and the principles will help them make a successful adaptation to others. In chronic illness, living this way will solve some illnesses. Illness can be a metaphor for disturbances in people's lives. The slang expression "I'm sick of this" may be truer than originally thought.

■ FEELINGS AND PHYSICAL PAIN

Some of my migraines are from fatigue, light, heat, noise, crowding, and other indignities. However, some are from painful thoughts and feelings that have somehow been translated into a very real physical pain in my eye. As I have applied these principles, the "painful thoughts and feelings" type of headache is mostly gone and the remaining ones may be caused by my neurology, not my relationships. Many other illnesses, especially stress related ones, may be ameliorated by living a more spiritual life.

Spiritual Well-Being and Relapse

Having achieved some spiritual well-being, people would like to keep going with their spiritual progress. Persevering with the spiritual principles, along with daily self-examination, keeps people well. All chronic illnesses are characterized by relapse. Spiritual well-being is also characterized by relapse into spiritual malaise. Without a frequent review of an adherence to spiritual principles, people are likely to lose ground. The link between spiritual relapse and physical relapse is the clearest in addictions. People who are working a Twelve Step program well can often hear a relapse approaching one of their peers by simply listening to them talk. A deterioration in spirituality comes shortly before the resumption of addictive drinking or drugging.

■ A STUPID AND ANNOYING WORLD

My own experience with addiction and spirituality is that if I live outside of this way of life for about two weeks, other people become stupid and annoying. It's unclear how the whole world knows to get stupid and annoying all at the same time, but they do. Or at least is seems that way. The reality is that my own spiritual state is relapsing, but part of that relapse is the denial of any responsibility for it.

Time and the Tenth Step

To protect against this type of relapse, the tenth Step of the Twelve Step programs reads: "We continued to take personal inventory and when we were wrong, promptly admitted it." We discover our fresh wrongs, we admit them, make amends for them, and move on. Doing this on a daily basis keeps the scale of wrongs small.

This is not a chore. Time spent in self-examination makes the rest of the day happier. People won't be persisting in patterns of thought and action that cause conflict with their Higher Power, themselves, and others. As an analogy, people don't usually resent the time spent in brushing their teeth because they like the way their mouths taste and feel when they brush. They don't ask, "Do I have to do it *every day*?" unless they are very young and childish. Similarly, people will feel better immediately when they do a daily moral inventory.

Paying Attention to the Present

Living a well examined life allows people the gift of mindfulness. They can afford to pay attention to their lives because they are not embarrassed about what they find. They can focus on the experience of living with color, sound, tastes, fun, friendships, work, and play. They don't have a need to manipulate life to accommodate their wrongs because they are free to live life.

This differs from the courage displayed in major spiritual self-examination. The major inventory was an examination of the past. People exhibit perseverance by examining their present. Both intentions and actions are inventoried. The areas of conflict in people's lives is examined. When it is their fault, they admit it, make amends, and change. When the fault belongs to other people, they try to change their behavior to adapt to or avoid the conflict, and accept the reality that other people may not change. This does not mean accepting victimization, but rather accepting that they have neither the right nor the power to force change in others. If they are abusive, others will need to get away from them. At this stage, people stop fighting wherever possible instead of collecting grievances and seeking revenge. People lose interest in the whole process of winning and losing and seek to "live and let live."

Power Outage

When people promptly admit their wrongs, others lose power. On the other hand, when people try to hide their wrongs, others gain power. People have to start guessing who noticed that they were wrong. In essence, they must prepare a cover story. They need to manipulate others to keep them from finding out or to shift the blame away from themselves. People require good memories so they can keep their stories straight.

By disclosing it all, people can't be pressured with the threat of revealing their secrets if they aren't actually a secret any more. In the Watergate scandal, it wasn't the burglary that got President Nixon in trouble, it was the cover up. In President Clinton's encounter with Monica Lewinsky, most people focused on his lying about his affair and trying to shift the blame, rather than the affair itself. If he had admitted it early in the process, it would have been hard to drag him all the way through the impeachment process.

A Daily Practice of Self-Restraint

Doing a daily personal inventory teaches self-restraint. They'll either learn to change or they'll be faced with the same problems in their inventory every day. It becomes a bit tedious to keep repeating the same wrongs, so people learn not to translate every discreditable thought into a regrettable action.

Looking at the Positive

A good way to take such an inventory is to make a daily inventory card that includes each of the spiritual principles defined in this book. People can take a negative inventory such as "How have I been dishonest?" "How have I lacked hope?" "How have I lacked courage?", and so on, but that can be a bit discouraging. It is more productive to do a positive inventory: "I was honest today, when I ..." "I was hopeful today, when I ..." "I displayed courage today when I ..." Even when people do such a positive inventory, their faults will come to them as they consider each principle they could have used.

The same method for daily inventory can be used to assess beliefs and actions about chronic illnesses. It's a good idea to persevere in self-examination by stating something like: "I am honest about my illness, as evidenced by ..." "I am hopeful in the face of my illness, as evidenced by..." "I have courage in the face of my illness, as evidenced by ..." and so on through these spiritual principles.

Like the longer inventory completed in the development of people's courage, this is an inventory of themselves, not of others. People avoid conclusions that they have done what they did because of others, and accept responsibility for all their actions, right or wrong. This may seem like a small point, but it is valuable. Instead of saying to someone "You make me angry!" they say "I am angry." Their anger is their own. What others have done may be the occasion of people's anger, but their anger is their own. Realizing that their feelings and actions are their own is the basis for aligning their thoughts, feelings, and actions with their principles.

It is important to inventory the good things people have done. People grow by building patterns of right conduct, rather than simply by eliminating what is wrong. They inventory how well they have set worthy goals and met them. They inventory how they have been a blessing to others in that day.

Doing a daily moral inventory helps people with decisions. A good decision making pattern is to keep an open mind as long as possible on any given topic or problem. This allows for maximum creativity. When minds are closed, danger is the result. If someone is jumping across a chasm, halfway across is not a good time to stop and wonder if they should have taken a longer running start. Instead, it's time to carry out the jump. After they have acted, they evaluate the results, and see where change is needed. This is a useful pattern for most decisions. While they're keeping an open mind, and considering all the possibilities, matching their possible behaviors with their daily moral inventory helps lead them to the right and useful choices.

Mid-Course Corrections

It is hard to make one set of decisions and have them all be right. People are much more likely to come to the right conclusions if they make preliminary decisions, carry them out, and then examine the results. Their examination will reveal the corrections needed. An airplane doesn't fly absolutely straight from one city to another. It heads off in the right direction and makes a whole series of mid-course corrections before arriving at its destination. Taking a daily moral inventory allows people to make mid-course corrections while they are still small and easily carried out.

Creating Both a Moral and Physical Inventory

In chronic illnesses, the patient often needs to take some form of daily inventory. The diabetic takes a blood sugar level. Those with circulatory disorders may take their blood pressure or pulse. Some with damaged hearts have artificial pacemakers to constantly correct an irregular heartbeat. People taking certain drugs need to check their blood levels of that drug, or have blood tests to see that the drug isn't causing damaging side effects. People on psychiatric medications get a "medication check" to see that it is still having the desired result. Small, mid-course corrections are crucial in the management of chronic illness. A moral inventory in the patient's mid-course corrections is just as important as including a physical inventory.

Perseverance is important for physicians and other clinicians, as well. Perseverance in addressing physical problems is a much more important requirement in the treatment of chronic illness than it is in the treatment of acute illness. In acute illness, the course of the treatment is likely to be short. Chronic illness can last the lifetime of the patient. Patience and perseverance are obvious requirements for those who want to do treatment well.

Perseverance in taking a personal inventory is a useful tool for the clinician to offer to the patient. Many health care providers are now doing a lifestyle inventory with their patients in terms of diet, exercise, stress, and allergies. This can be extended to include these spiritual principles in the lifestyle inventory. How has the patient been honest, hopeful, faithful, courageous, and so on, and so forth. The areas of life in which the patient is not acting according to spiritual principles are likely to be the areas of major stress.

Perseverance: A Useful Tool

Perseverance in taking a personal inventory is a useful tool for clinicians in their own practice. Every spiritual principle used in this book is as useful for the art of medicine as it is for the treatment of illness. Clinicians can ask themselves, as they review their professional conduct for the day, "How have I been honest with patients, staff, third parties?" "I cannot disclose that information due to patient confidentiality" is an honest answer that can also be used. The italicized words that follow in the questions below show the principles underlying the Twelve Steps. These questions should be asked frequently to keep on track

"How have I had *hope* and demonstrated it to my patients?"

"How have I had *faith* in a Higher Power (which need not be God) and shown that faith in my work?"

"How have I practiced medicine with *courage* today?"

"How have I had *integrity*, and shown others how to have it?"

"How have I been *willing* to be guided and changed?"

"How have I had *humility* and shown it in my personal interactions?"

"How have I demonstrated *compassion* for others and myself?"

"How have I been *just* and fair in my dealings?"

"How well have I *persevered* in practicing these principles and in continuing to treat the chronic illness patient well?"

"How have I been aware of my *Higher Power* today?"

"How have I been of *service*?"

Growing in Love and Fellowship

As people continue to take their personal inventory, they will do less damage to their relationships with their Higher Power, themselves, and others. They will do more to grow in love and fellowship and their inner chaos will fade, and serenity will be the end result. This inventory is a form of conscious contact with themselves, allowing them to be fully present to God, themselves, and others.

Suggestions for perseverance in your life and work:

- Continue to take your own inventory, and when you are wrong, promptly admit it. This includes moral wrongs as well as mistakes.
- Practice self-care, so that you are physically, mentally, emotionally, and spiritually capable of perseverance.
- Encourage patients to accept that there will be good days and bad days, and to make the most of the good days and rest on the bad days.
- Ask your patients to do a daily reflection on what they have done each day to make their own life better and to better the lives of those around them.

Bowen F. White

> Even the fool who persists in his folly will become wise.
>
> William Blake

A True Model of Perseverance

The poet William Blake was certainly a model of perseverance. He had a way of seeing, a vision that he pursued regardless of the sacrifices that were required. His ability to honor the creative impulse within and allow that impulse to determine the trajectory of his life was remarkable. It did not result in material wealth. For most of his life he had trouble rubbing two shillings together. But as he lay in his deathbed he was composing songs to the angels that surrounded him. His return on investment was ecstasy on earth.

As a spiritual principle, perseverance qualifies because much of what people get from culture functions as a distraction from targeting the knot. The culture in the US supports a certain kind of perseverance in attaining the American dream. Everyone who went through medical school and specialty training needed that perseverance to make it through. Perseverance indeed, but the longer the training the narrower the area of expertise and the greater the level of technical competence. The return on investment is a sizable enhancement in personal wealth. Those that endure it, deserve it. Perseverance pays.

Medical doctors worked long, hard hours. Doctors felt they deserved something tangible since having something to show for it is the most important part of the American dream. As doctors, they have those initials in front of their names "to show for it." This relentless drive toward a goal can be carried out without the influence of spiritual values. It is easy to become disconnected from a spiritual reference point. But once again, illness may jolt them awake and aid them in realignment with what is most important in their lives. Just as it has with some patients/clients, it isn't necessary to wait to get sick in order to reconnect. People can reconnect daily, hourly, in the next thought, after the next thought, or before the next thought. People can do this through spiritual practice. Practice does help them remember, reconnect, and experience perfect love.

■ THE STRENGTH OF PRAYER AND SPIRITUAL READING

A routine that author Don Campbell used seems helpful to me. Don would get up every morning and spend one hour in prayer and spiritual reading. He would then walk briskly for one hour. That was his practice. And as he walked he would set up a rhythm between his steps and the seven words of the Jesus prayer: "Lord Jesus Christ have mercy on me." His intention was to eventually get to the place where this Eastern Orthodox prayer would be a perpetual mantra in his comings and goings throughout the day. By focusing on those words he was repeating the name of God and asking for mercy. But I don't think what he was doing was only that. Even the words "God" and "mercy" are concepts. What I think Don was doing was consciously creating an opening for God to use to break through, past the words and manifest. Meister Eckart, a 13th century mystical Christian who eventually was kicked out of the catholic church posthumously, said that we have to let go of our concept of God for God.

I think that is what Don Campbell was doing. That prayer is a centering prayer. As spiritual practice goes, that prayer had been used for ages to help one center and then enter the heart of God. The idea being that the words take us into a certain psychospiritual space where we can experience the presence of God.

The way Don described his early morning prayer experience was like sitting in a waiting room. He would imagine that he was sitting in God's waiting room every morning. He would be there waiting just in case God had something to say to him. Sometimes God had some message to convey, sometimes not. But Don wanted to be available there daily, in the waiting room, just in case. That was his practice. After his morning prayer and exercise ritual he usually met with someone at a local cafe for a breakfast chat. The topic usually included something consistent with the spiritual journey. If it was not initially, it was eventually. He had a way of visiting with others that would clarify the situation by seeing it in the light of a spiritual flash-light. The issue could be addressed from a values reference point that allowed decisions to be made in alignment with one's highest values. He never tried to stuff any ideas down people's throats at breakfast, or any other time for that matter. But he would be available as a mirror to reflect back to others what they were pondering as he dialogued with them. He used the term "dialogue" and defined it as a meeting of meanings. Meaning was central to Don. That was his quest in conversation with others. What is the meaning for them to derive from having to face this issue now in their lives? I do not want to make it sound as though a conversation with Don was always very heavy, very serious. To the contrary. His energy was always light. He had a great sense of humor and a wonderful ability to laugh at him-self. Some say laughter is the best medicine. My friend, Patch Adams says that friendship is the best medicine. Regardless, when you put the two together they are very important tools for persevering on the road to wholeness. Suffice to say that Don Campbell was a model of perseverance, a model inclusive of the joy that one experi-ences during and following one's spiritual practice.

For Don it was not only a matter of the inward journey, but also the outward journey. Action in the world was enhanced by his non-action. The time he spent centering helped him remember and reconnect so that in his dealings in the field of action, the pressures of the world were less likely to coerce him into unhealthy responses. His practice helped him keep his eye focused on the knot when the world and its stresses wanted his head turned elsewhere.

■ THE PRAYER OF THE FROG

I was recently in Germany to speak at a meeting sponsored by an association dedicated to the treatment of the whole person. I had been in Europe with Patch Adams. A movie of the same name starring Robin Williams had opened in the United States on Christmas day 1998. He and I had traveled there to open the movie in five European cities in March of 1999. While in Germany with people that Patch had known for years who were responsible for the German premier, a conversation ensued. In that conversation, Patch suggested that they use me as a speaker at one of their meetings. It so happened that one of their speakers had canceled. I was asked to fill in for the absent presenter. I returned to Germany to open the meeting.

When I was there a couple of folks from Fordam University were there to speak also. I never met them, but sensed from the meeting materials that they were connected to the work of Anthony de Mello, a Jesuit Priest who spent much of his life in India. In the campus bookstore I purchased some of de Mello's books. In one of the books is an excellent example of perseverance. In the book, "The Prayer of the Frog" is a tale about a printing block displayed in Kyoto, Japan at the Obaku Monastery. The story goes like this: there was a Japanese student of Zen named Tetsugen who decided to take on the task of printing thousands of copies of the sutras in his language. He traveled throughout Japan collecting money for the project. Until then the sutras were only available in Chinese. He thanked all contributors equally regardless of the size of their contribution. After 10 years he had what he needed. But, just then, a natural disaster in the form of a flood inundated the people. He spent all the funds he had collected to help the flood victims.

So, he began again. He spent years collecting the required funds. Just as he had enough money, an epidemic struck. Tetsugen spent all those monies in support of the epidemic victims. Once more he began again. After 20 years of effort, he had succeeded in his task. The printing block that produced that first edition is now on display in Kyoto, Japan at the Obaku Monastery. Japanese parents tell their children that Tetsugen made three editions of the sutras. The first two editions were invisible "and far superior to the third." Tetsugen demonstrated perseverance. On the way to his goal he never lost sight of the knot. And his most superior work came on the way there.

Ways in which you might use perseverance to enhance your relationships with the chronically ill include:

- Being in the medical field requires perseverance. You had it, but what do you do when you run out of juice? Pray. Pray for the juice.
- Let go of having to control the patient. Let your values be the lighthouse and give you direction.

- Perseverance could be resting in God. Even God rested. On the seventh day he rested. Rest when you need to rest. It will help you persevere.
- Follow the principles. Perceive power as lamb power, not as a way to manipulate others. Help other people support us in our perseverance when we are in the face of difficulty.

REFERENCE

1. S. Mitchell, *Tao Te Ching, a New English Version*, Harper Collins, New York, 1992, p. 79.

14
Chapter Fourteen

Principle 11: Spiritual Awareness
John A. Mac Dougall

> This noble eightfold path ... right views, right aspirations,
> right speech, right conduct, right livelihood, right effort, right
> mindfulness, and right contemplation.
> Dhammacakkappavattanasutta, verse 4, *The Pali Canon*,
> *c.* 250 B.C.

Step Eleven and the Spiritual Awareness Principle

The Eleventh Step is: "Sought through prayer and meditation to improve our conscious contact with God, as we understood him, praying only for knowledge of His will for us and power to carry that out."

Connecting with Self and Others Through Prayer and Meditation

Principle 11 builds on the concept of perseverance. It allows people to get in conscious contact with themselves. People use all twelve of the spiritual principles to become the finest version of themselves that they can be. Having restored their relationships with themselves and others, they now turn to their Higher Power to make sure they continue and develop the conscious contact they have made. They are aware of their own conduct and their relationships with others through their spiritual self-examination. The Eleventh Step gives people the chance to be aware of their relationships with their Higher Power through prayer and meditation.

After people have made self-examination part of their daily lives, they then complete the process by including prayer and meditation. As they begin to use self-examination instead of self-absorption, they naturally include other people and their Higher Power in their thoughts. As a result, they develop a rhythm: self-examination first, then prayer that arises out of their self-discovery, followed by meditation on the nature of their Higher Power's will for them.

Opening Up to Guidance

In the face of chronic illness, people need to be open to a variety of outcomes for their lives, ranging from a cure to death. As long as they have determined the right outcome and insist on it, they are not open to guidance. They are still applying their own will to the situation and hoping for the best.

> ### ■ THE IMPORTANCE OF CONSCIOUS CONTACT
>
> Spiritual awareness needs to include conscious contact with a Higher Power, not just a belief about a Higher Power. I believe many things that don't matter. For example, I believe that Beijing is the capital of China. I don't have any reason to doubt this fact, but it really doesn't matter to me. After all, I haven't been there and I don't know anyone there. I have no relationship with it. For a Higher Power belief to matter, I need a relationship, and I need to be in touch.

Conscious contact with a Higher Power is a lot like conscious contact with other people. People might have all kinds of friends, but for them to be more than a memory they need to talk and really listen to them. People might have beliefs about a Higher Power, but for those beliefs to have any real impact on their lives, they need to talk to their Higher Power and listen for the guidance.

■ PRAYER DEVELOPMENT

People can talk to their Higher Power any way they want. They need not learn a specialized style of prayer to do so. My original home is New York City where a local proverb goes: "The more you complain, the longer God lets you live." Even complaint is a form of communication. Perhaps it's not the noblest, but it gets people started. Their form of prayer can mature as the person advances in development.

Taking Prayers Literally

When Alan D. was little, his mother taught him the child's prayer "Now I lay me down to sleep. I pray the Lord my soul to keep. If I die before I wake, I pray the Lord my soul to take." Then she would return when she was drunk and beat him. He took that prayer literally and would ask God to let him die. When that didn't happen, he would feel as abandoned by God as he did by his mother. He gave up prayer for many years on the theory that it didn't work. When he began to hear of the value of prayer in recovery, he resumed praying. Today he prays in the manner of this spiritual principle: instead of using prayer to inform God of his will, he prays to know and do the will of God. It is working well for him.

Knowledge and Power

There are many times in people's lives when they have had the knowledge of what to do, but just lacked the power to carry it out. Now when they pray for knowledge, they pray for power as well. Having a Higher Power doesn't mean giving up their power, it means getting more power by aligning themselves with this Higher Power. To do so, they avoid placing limitations on God. They don't pray with terms and conditions. Instead, they may tell their Higher Power what they want, think, and feel. They do their best to abandon the impulse of telling God how to best provide for them. Instead they ask for guidance and the ability to do the right thing.

Questioning God

A desire to question God is natural. People often wonder why things are the way they are. They wish God would give them the answers. A more mature spirituality involves understanding that people are the ones being questioned by life. Instead of demanding answers about life, people come to realize that they are being asked by life to answer how they will live when faced with their evolving circumstances. Instead of asking God "why me?" when faced with chronic illness, they learn to ask themselves the following questions: "What meaning can I find in this?" "How will I behave towards others?" and "How can I be of service to my fellow human beings?" In his book *Man's Ultimate Search for Meaning,*[1] Victor Frankl writes: "We need to stop asking ourselves about the meaning of life, and to think of ourselves as those who were being questioned by life, daily and hourly. Everything can be taken away from man but one thing—to choose one's attitude in a given set of circumstances, to choose one's own way."

■ **EXPLORING DIFFERENT TYPES OF PRAYERS**

There have been many times in my life I have asked God to remove my headaches. I have been particularly vocal when in pain. I cannot report any progress from those prayers. Although I believe that God could relieve my pain, it is clear that He has not done so. That particular type of prayer simply wasn't working well. Today, I ask God to give me an awareness of what to do, minute by minute, and to give me the power to live well: at peace with myself, others, and with God. That seems to work much better. This way my headaches don't give other people headaches, real or figurative.

In addition, I have been able to coach some addicts and alcoholics who have chronic pain. We talk about how to live with pain and also about non-addictive methods of pain relief. Living gracefully relieves pain. At first, it does so because we aren't creating more. Then it does so as we give up struggling against the pain. Our help continues as we develop acceptance of life the way it really is, and finally find enthusiasm for it.

Listening and Talking

Prayer can be either talking aloud or it can take place only in people's minds. Meditation is listening. People listen to themselves, to other people, to their Higher Power, and to life itself. Meditating on their own words, reflecting on what they have said and done is a tool for change, much like spiritual self-examination. Meditation at the end of the day gives people a chance to understand and find meaning in the day's events. This practice proves to be valuable to people especially as they grow older. There comes a time, towards the end of life, when people's memories become a greater source of pleasure than their future plans. If they've been reflecting on their lives along the way, they will be well guided and are likely to have much to be satisfied for when looking back over their lives.

People can read worthwhile literature and meditate on it. Hazelden and other publishers create a wide range of meditation books, all for different populations. Many people find a daily reading a good basis for meditation. Others will meditate on a scripture passage. One method is to take a story from religious literature and meditate on it from the point of view of each of the characters in the story.

A Walk in the Woods

Others choose to meditate on nature and on life itself. The Buddhist idea of mindfulness is useful here. Instead of sleepwalking through life, people can be mindful of their lives right now. How hot or cold is it? What are their emotions? What does the air feel like and how lightly or heavily does it weigh on them? They can be mindful of the colors and textures of what they see. They can contemplate their structures, and see life where it exists. One method used at Hazelden is a meditation walk, in which a group of patients walk slowly and silently through the woods. The goal is to discover how much can be seen, heard, and felt, and to be open to whatever their Higher Power has for them. The discussions that take place following the walks are usually filled with enthusiasm and insight.

Take a Deep Breath

People can meditate on their physical lives as well. Many meditation techniques include a focus on breathing. Progressive muscular relaxation and a systematic desensitization to anxiety are forms of meditation on the interplay between body and mind. Some cancer patients are using visualization in an effort to combat tumors. They visualize themselves free of disease. Even if it doesn't reduce the cancer, it allows the person to relax and be less under the control of the illness.

■ RELEASING TENSION

I discovered that I was tensing up in response to migraine pain. It feels like protection, but it actually makes things worse. By letting go and relaxing, the pain gets briefly worse, and then it subsides to a significant degree.

People may choose to meditate to music or nature sounds. There are a number of recording companies that combine classical music and nature sounds. I personally prefer instrumental music. My favorite meditative piece is the "Meditation" from Jules Massenet's opera *Thais* in a 1968 Berlin Philharmonic recording.[2] I lie down with a cloth blindfold for darkness and listen to the violin solo. In this meditation, I imagine that the violin represents my spirit. The dense orchestral passages represent the noise and confusion of life.

Sometimes the solo violin disappears, and then it appears again, and at the end of the piece, they are peacefully resolved.

Combining Meditation and Prayer

Meditating on the will of their Higher Power is the perfect complement to prayer. Having asked for knowledge of God's will and the power to carry it out, people need to listen. A quiet time with an open mind and spirit proves valuable. Answers may appear at that moment or perhaps later. What was once the occasional flash of intuition becomes a regular dialogue with their Higher Power. Answers sometimes come in what people hear from a trusted friend, in a meeting, a book, or from within themselves. Some people hear their own voice coming from somewhere within, but suddenly the ideas are fresh and new. This can be their Higher Power giving them back what they need. It is useful to check out this voice and its messages with a spiritual guide or trusted friend, to make sure it's not just a distortion of their own will.

A Sense of Belonging

The disciplines of prayer and meditation become natural. They become a reflexive part of life, instead of being work to be done. As people become spiritually aware, they are naturally centered within themselves and guided by a Higher Power. Alcoholics Anonymous (A.A.) gives people an account of this peace and serenity: "Perhaps one of the greatest rewards of meditation and prayer is the sense of belonging that comes to us. We no longer live in a completely hostile world. We are no longer lost and frightened and purposeless. The moment we catch even a glimpse of God's will, the moment we begin to see truth, justice, and love as real and eternal things in life, we are no longer deeply disturbed by all the seeming evidence to the contrary that surrounds us in purely human affairs. We know that God lovingly watches over us. We know that when we turn to Him, all will be well with us, here and hereafter."[3]

Having put spiritual principles into practice, and become centered, people are now ready to move onto Step Twelve and begin to provide the greatest possible service to others. The journey continues as people progress in their spiritual growth. Meanwhile, this growth ensures their own progress by giving away what they have received.

Suggestions for spiritual awareness in your life and work:

- Seek through prayer and meditation to have conscious contact with God as you understand God. Pray for knowledge of the next right thing to do and the power to do it.
- One possible prayer for the end of your day is, "God, I'm going to bed now. They're your patients, take care of them."
- Offer to pray for and with your patients.
- Encourage patients to pray for themselves and others.
- Teach meditation techniques, for conscious contact with their Higher Power, for positive imaging of health, for relaxation, and for pain relief.

Bowen F. White

There is a medicine that heals the healer
A practice that creates a healing environment
In which the great physician moves
It is not taught at the university
But by the universe
It is a sacred practice
A sacrament to the one life that binds you to me
No one can hang its mark upon the wall
No one can claim the franchise
Saying, "I am the one who knows"
We all know in our not knowing
The inner wounds speak through the body
Listening past the words one hears
The inner voice calling saying, "touch me here, this is where I
   suffer."
I want to enter that room
I want to touch that place
And attend the birth of a child of God
Into awareness
That is healing to us both.

Bowen White

There is no doubt that awareness has to be a spiritual principal because without it people lose their balance. They fall off the metaphorical rope. Spiritual awareness may be redundant because when people are aware, they are awake. They are present to the possibilities of the moment. They are caught in the moment, without the distraction of past or future. They are able to make healthy choices that help them deal with the reality of now. And being present, in the now, is a spiritual practice.

This story illustrates the point nicely: The student asked the teacher if one becomes divine upon attaining enlightenment. The teacher was silent. The student fell asleep while awaiting a reply. At their next lesson the student asked again. The teacher was again silent. Once again, the student fell asleep. When they met again, the student asked anew if one became divine upon reaching enlightenment. The student was becoming drowsy when the teacher finally replied, "No." The student was startled by his teacher's voice and asked, "what does one become?" "Awake," the teacher replied. Of course, it also means being present without expectations or assumptions.

The Joys of Respect and Consideration

Anthony de Mello in his book, *Prayer of the Frog*,[4] tells a story about making an assumption that may actually make people more aware and more awake. The story goes like this: A guru was sitting in meditation in his cave when the abbot of a famous monastery came to visit. When the guru asked as to the cause of the visit the abbot told him a troubled tale. The monastery, once well known and flourishing had fallen into dire straits. The few monks that remained were anything but joyful in their practice. The abbot then wanted to know the cause of the fall of his prominent monastery. The guru said that the cause was ignorance. "Ignorance of what?" queried the abbot. "One of your number is the Messiah in disguise and you are ignorant of this," the guru replied and then returned to his reverie. The abbot was filled with excitement as he traveled back to his home. The Messiah had chosen his humble monastery for his earthly abode. What a blessing that such an event would come into the life of all those there. But who could it be? Since the Messiah was in disguise, it could be anyone. But, all the monks had defects so how could any of them be the perfect one? Of course, defects could help hide the truth of the Messiah's identity. Defects are part of the disguise!

Upon returning, the abbot relayed the story to the monks of his visit to the guru and his new revelation. The monks were amazed and excited. Who among them was the Messiah? It was incredible that one in their midst was the One that the world was awaiting. The disguise would have to be so good that no one would be able to penetrate through to the truth. Therefore, anyone could be the perfect one.

The outcome? Everyone began to treat everyone else with the most respect and consideration. After all, the person to whom they were relating could be the Messiah in disguise. The energy and atmosphere in the monastery went from dour to joyful. Soon the monastery was attracting aspirants and bristling with renewal "—and once again the Church reechoed with the holy and joyful chant of monks who were aglow with the spirit of Love."

Growing Young

A cultural anthropologist named Ashley Montagu who taught at Princeton wrote a truly remarkable book *Growing Young*[5] (now out of print). He states that people are not meant to grow into the kind of grownups they become. They are not supposed to grow old, they are instead to grow young. He uses strong scholarship to support his view that people are meant to stay in a developmental process throughout the life cycle. Thus, people are to be continuously unfolding their potential, as opposed to stopping development once their vocation can support their lifestyle. Montagu's definition of health is the ability to love, work, play, and think soundly. Through awareness, people can think soundly. Without awareness, they cannot. Most of what people do, they do out of habit. That includes their thinking. Their habitual patterns of thought are culturally driven. They have to wake up, to become aware that what has happened to them has set them up to be externally focused and internally neglectful. Their point of reference is not a spiritual knot. Their collective feelings of inadequacy are reinforced by advertising and placated by consumption. People are told what to buy to make them whole, complete, and fulfilled.

The "fix" of consumption, of consumerism is a remedy that exploits their low feelings for themselves. People become addicted to any "fix" that lets them cope with those bad feelings and feel better. People become fearful and anxious without their medicine.

People are full of fear that someone may find out the truth about them. Before people can think soundly they have to examine their thinking. When people were small, were they actually encouraged to question the authority figures in their lives? Weren't they told to respect authority? It wasn't just their parents. It was all the grown-ups, clergy included—especially the clergy. The clergy spoke with the ultimate authority. Who could possibly question that? Could it be . . . Satan? Talk about instilling the fear of God. To question was to open themselves to Satan's thoughts, Satan's thinking. Go with the program, don't make waves and they'll be safe with them, the chosen ones.

The Power of Early Programming

Do they know any of the research that demonstrates just how powerful early programming is, at least with cats? Kittens are born with their eyes shut. And if those kittens are raised in an environment in which horizontal lines and surfaces are the only lines and surfaces present, certain, repeatable results ensue. When the kittens open their eyes they learn to see the world as it is present around them. And that world is a horizontal world. They adapt and learn to function in that world rather nicely, doing what cats do outside of their natural environment. But, when those same cats are placed in an environment that contains vertical structures, problems arise. The cats have learned to see their world in a certain way, horizontal. Their way of thinking about their world worked for them before.

They are limited by that world view that wasn't reality based. And in the larger scheme of things which includes the vertical perspective they encounter difficulty. When they encounter a vertical structure they bump into it because they cannot see anything but horizontal structures. They continue to bump into stuff that they have not learned to perceive. They filter out what does not fit with their database of perceptual biases. They are not stupid. They are doing their best.

Think about how parents treat their children. Often, they want to protect them. Isn't that what kids want from their parents? But, what they have learned and how they have learned to think may not serve them well when their horizontal biases confront vertical experience. Today, those children are grown up. They can be doing their best and doing things well to demonstrate their competence so that they will not be seen as inadequate.

> "People compelled by craving crawl like snared rabbits."
> Dhammapada, 24.9

People cannot think soundly when they are not aware that they are "snared rabbits." People with overt problems like a chronic illness may use that world stopping event to begin their movement to freedom. The problem is, their programming sets them up to want to find the "fix" to get them back the way they were before they got sick. Clinicians, at least, are trained to do this. But, by doing this, they may be helping the patients stay stuck. What clinicians can choose to do, although it may feel uncomfortable, is to serve as an instrument for the patients to use in the exploration of the ultimate questions. That doesn't mean that clinicians shouldn't use their clinical acumen in the service of their patients. Clinicians need to do that and more. They cannot do the "more" until they become free themselves. Clinicians cannot break free alone. They need something greater than themselves to assist them in the process of getting unsnarled. The abbot needed council from the guru to create a truly sacred space in a place where culture says it is a given. He used someone in his support community to get his balance back and refocus on the knot. The guru helped him wake up and see the familiar in a new way.

The Divine Presence Inside

Just holding in awareness that there is a divine presence inside, inside everyone, changes the way people use their gifts and energy. Whatever people can do to maintain that awareness or get it back when they are lost or forget, serves to render a more balanced view. Think of the horizontal perspective as cultural conditioning. People cannot ignore the horizontal view of culture as they do have an ego that continues to function in that world. This is the realm of the scared person inside who is driven by fear and resistant to change. The horizontal line can be seen here as a minus sign, and there is concern that people, at any moment, can be discovered as inadequate. So people must be constantly vigilant as they defend the image that they want the world to have for them. People are defensive, yet quick to deny it when someone gets too close to the truth. And if people can no longer deny, they will rationalize their behavior to validate staying the course, even though they have clearly lost their way.

People need the balance provided by vertical awareness to get back, or stay, on course. Sure they have a scared one inside, bound by culture, driven by fear who is resistant to change and who deals with discomfort through unhealthy, though normal, coping behaviors. But that is not the whole story. That is an unbalanced view of humanity. People also have a sacred one inside that is not culture bound, who is open to being vulnerable, defenseless, and who seeks to change him/herself through love in a community of friends who seek change as well.

It is the vertical perspective or the spiritual view that provides the needed balance so people can be in the world with its overwhelming problems, and not be overwhelmed. On the local level, the connection to something greater than their little, false or scared self is necessary to keep from falling off course on their own healing journey. Honoring the divinity of self and others by paying attention to the vertical domain provides the energy required to risk doing the right thing even when others don't.

But that loving community of support that reminds people of the sacredness of each person from the vertical perspective, often functions at odds with the dominant culture. Then, when people begin to do the things they need to do to be healthy, even people within their own church, or temple, or, for that matter, that are in their own family may wonder what is wrong with them. When people are different, more authentic and perhaps more willing to rock the boat, that can be very unsettling to some of the other passengers on board.

Patients may choose to have their clinicians help them deal with that conflict. But, whom do the clinicians have? And whom do their patients have to provide them with healthy support outside of their relationship with their clinician? The importance of healthy support keeps cropping up. God uses people, people with awareness, the vertical awareness that they are here to serve. In the next chapter the spiritual principle of service will be explored.

Ways to enhance your life and create meaningful relationships with the chronically ill through spiritual awareness might include:

- Encourage your patients to play. After all, play is a form of spiritual awareness. Take the first step by going to an elementary school and participating in recess. Encourage them to look for the radiance in the children's eyes and then take the time to reflect on what age they quit being radiant.
- In your practice and in everyday life, it is important to remember that everyone is a God holder. We are all children of God and should be treated accordingly.
- In your practice, quit focusing on giving what you think your patient's deserve. Don't withhold warmth regardless of how they treat you.
- Spirituality is not somber and heavy. It is about being a child, being caring, full of life, buoyant, and playful. It's about living fully in the moment.

REFERENCES

1. Frankl, V., Hunt, S., et al., *Man's Ultimate Search For Meaning*, Insight Books, 1997.
2. "Adagio Karajan," Deutsche Grammophon 445 282-2 GH, 1999.
3. *Twelve Steps and Twelve Traditions*, Alcoholics Anonymous World Services, New York, 1953, p. 105.
4. Anthony de Mello, *Prayer of the Frog*, revised edition, Doubleday, New York, 1998.
5. Ashley Montagu, *Growing Young*, McGraw-Hill, New York, 1981.

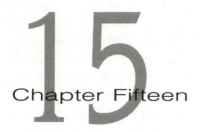

Chapter Fifteen

Principle 12: Service

John A. Mac Dougall

Whoever destroys a single life is as guilty as though he had destroyed the entire world; and whoever rescues a single life earns as much merit as though he had rescued the entire world.

Mishna, Sanhedrin

Step Twelve and the Service Principle

The Twelfth Step is: "Having had a spiritual awakening as the result of these steps, we tried to carry this message to alcoholics, and to practice these principles in all our affairs."

The Meaning of Service

Service is usually understood as something done for others. It is also something people do for themselves, their happiness, well-being, and spiritual growth. In their development of spiritual awareness, they asked their Higher Power to give them knowledge and power. A major part of their purpose is to be of service to others.

Humans are not well prepared for independence. In modern society they are interdependent for nearly everything: food, clothing, shelter, medical care, love, friendship, and recovery. If their interdependence consists only of an even exchange of goods and services in a market based economy, it is hard for the human race as a whole to progress. To get beyond merely being even, many of them will need to be of service.

An Opportunity for Sharing

A result of a spiritual awakening might include the conclusion that people are accompanied through life by a Higher Power with whom they are able to achieve that which they could never do alone. This spiritual awakening is a gift that comes with a purpose: the opportunity to pass it onto others. If they are not willing to pass on the love and help they have received, they may not be able to keep it for themselves. Hoarding makes everyone poorer, giving makes everyone richer.

■ THE SERVICE CONCEPT AND A.A.

The concept of service is obvious in addiction and recovery. In 1935, when Bill Wilson, the co-founder of A.A., went looking for another drunk in Akron, Ohio, he went primarily to keep himself sober. While he was unable to stay sober directly, he intuited that if he tried to help another drunk, he himself would be able to stay sober. He was right. The message of the Twelfth Step is that there is hope for a good life. By practicing all twelve of the spiritual principles no matter what, regardless of the circumstances of life, life becomes good. Service to others is one of these important principles, and provides a forum for the expression of the others.

■ SERVICE: A WINDING PATH TO HAPPINESS

Roy Campanella, a patient at New York University Hospital, was serving others by visiting from room to room and giving hope. In boosting other people's morale he was improving his own. People who help others, in any form, often report that they are getting more than they give both in satisfaction and happiness. It is difficult to be happy directly, but it comes as a by-product of other things. Service is a roundabout path to happiness.

■ SERVING GOD

Years ago, I visited a hospice in India that was run by Mother Theresa's order of nuns. The admissions criteria was simple: if you have any-where else to go, go there. The hospice was located in an old ware-house, full of dying people on little metal beds. The patients seemed relatively happy. I attributed that to being well loved and cared for. The nuns who worked there seemed very happy and serene as well. I asked one, "Why are you so happy?" She replied, "Because we have Jesus as our guest every day. Wouldn't you be happy?" In serving others, she was serving God and bringing joy into her own life.

The Great Joy in Life

The greatest joy in life is to be of genuine and valuable service to others. This becomes more true as people age and consider their mortality. The desire to make a difference becomes stronger.

■ HERE ON EARTH TO SERVE OTHERS

My enjoyment of my work with chemically dependent patients comes from those times when I make a difference. The medallion that I received at the end of a Hazelden training program reads: "We are here on earth to serve others." My hope for this book is not that it will be great literature, but that it will be useful to those who read it.

"Enough" Never Seems to Come

One barrier to this spiritual principle is the idea that people have to take care of their own emotional and financial security first. After they have enough love and money they will be free to serve. However, "enough" never seems to come as long as people remain self-centered. Before people have their spirituality they tend to love things and use people. As they mature and grow, they love people and use things. If they still believe that the world owes them a living, the living they have is never good enough. If they come to believe that they owe the world their ideas, effort, and themselves in service to others, they become happy. They develop the passion that comes with being a player in life instead of a spectator. Generosity is good treatment for self-absorption, and as they become generous people, the impact of their problems diminishes.

Governance as a Form of Service

One way to begin to be more service oriented is to think of governance as a form of service. There are many situations that call for people to take some form of governance. People may govern by being managers or supervisors at work, leaders in organizations, or parents to their children. If leaders think of governance as getting other people to do their will, then their days will be full of conflict. If leaders focus on getting others to do their will, other people will be free to focus on evading the leaders' will, and both find themselves on the road to stalemate. If, instead, leaders think of their responsibilities for governance as a form of service to others, they will go forward in a much better spirit, and encounter less resistance.

If parents believe that parenting consists of getting their children to "mind," then the parents will always be disappointed that they do not "mind" perfectly. If they believe that parenting is to be of service to their children by teaching them adult skills, they will be pleased as their children grow in ability and self-control. If supervisors believe that supervising employees consists of getting them to do what they want, they will be like frustrated parents at work. If supervisors believe that supervising employees consists of serving others by supplying resources and coaching them for success, they will usually respond well. Those who don't respond to encouragement usually have made a commitment to discouragement, out of their own lack of spiritual progress. Love and tolerance is still the best action.

■ THE "FLOWER CHART"

I have been a pastor of Methodist churches for over 17 years. Most churches have an elected member who is in charge of flowers. If this person envisions this responsibility solely as governance, there is conflict. If someone brings unscheduled flowers that aren't on the "flower chart" this becomes a problem that only can be solved by shaming the person into not doing it again.

On the other hand, if the member in charge of flowers envisions the job as service, and someone brings unscheduled flowers, it's no problem. The member simply finds another vase, adds water and flowers, finds a place for them in church, and informs the pastor as to whom they should thank during the announcements. It's no problem at all. Service works better than mere governance in every area of leadership, both great or small.

The *Tao Te Ching* includes a poem about service:

When the Master governs, the people
are hardly aware that he exists.
Next best is a leader who is loved.
Next, one who is feared.
The worst is one who is despised.

If you don't trust the people,
you make them untrustworthy.

The Master doesn't talk, he acts.
When his work is done,
the people say, "Amazing:
we did it, all by ourselves!"[1]

Finding the Right Balance

If people have chosen to develop their spiritual awareness through prayer and meditation, they have invited their Higher Power to work through them. God will serve others through their service. Spirituality consists of their relationships with Higher Power, self, and others. Service aligns them in a right relationship with all three.

Being of service improves health. Altruism is the belief system in which people respond to life's stresses with service to others. In a study of the impact of mature emotional defenses on health, 4.3 percent of 55-year-old men with mature emotional defenses, such as altruism, sublimation, and humor became chronically ill during the next five years. A total of 14.5 percent of the 55-year-old men with immature emotional defenses such as: projection, passive aggression, acting out, and fantasy, became chronically ill during the next five years.[2] Improved health, relationships, and spirituality all result from serving others.

A Rich Opportunity to Live a New Way of Life

Many principles have been introduced throughout the course of this book. It would be natural for someone to look at the list and despair. A different approach should be taken instead of asking how all the work can be done, Look at the principles not as work to be done, but as an opportunity to live a life that is easier and more fun than the old way of life. Instead of working at these principles, they can be experimented with, in a spirit of curiosity and openness to change. After all, these principles are not things to do, they are things to be and become.

Suggestions for service in your life and work:

- Having had a spiritual awakening of your own as the result of these steps, carry a message of hope to others, and practice these principles in all your affairs.
- Cultivate gratitude for the calling to service, and keep the focus on your calling to serve others.
- Share your experience, strength, and hope with patients and colleagues.
- Encourage patients to be of service to others, within the limitations imposed by their illnesses.
- Tell patients when their lives and their actions are of service to you.
- Encourage patients to examine how living according to these spiritual principles could improve their quality of life.

Bowen F. White

> Act as if everything depended on you, and trust as if everything
> depended on God.
>
> > St. Ignatius

There is something here that has to do with the spiritual principle of service. There is some action that is required of clinicians, yet they have to let go of their concern for the results of that action. Therefore, clinicians must trust that God is the designated driver and where things end up is the right place. There is some action in the world, that is uniquely theirs to do. There is something that clinicians are called to do that represents the way that they can best serve the common good. That "something to do" reminds them of what is most important for their own healing. Their patients, regardless of their illness, need this as well. Unfortunately, no one else can tell clinicians what that calling is. If they hear the call and align attention and energy to act on that call, they must trust that the designated driver will get them home. People take action and surrender simultaneously. When people are drunk with God in this way the ego's intoxicants are like dry land to a fish. Their old behaviors are put aside as they relax into being their true self in the service of the common good. Trusting that God can use them to do something positive for the community in spite of their ineptness, they take action in the form of service.

Martin Luther King, Jr. says that the most urgent and persistent life question is: "what are you doing for someone else?" That is a good question. Another equally good question is, "why are you doing what you're doing for others?" The following story best illustrates this theory.

In 1980, a woman named Evy Macdonald got sick. Evy was a nurse and found herself in the intensive care unit that she had formerly run. Her body quit working and she was undergoing a workup by a neurologist to determine the cause of her malfunction. Things were heading downhill quickly to the extent that they were trying to talk her into going on to a ventilator due to her poor respiratory function.

Finally, her neurologist came in to give her an update on her condition. He looked out the window as he proceeded to tell Evy that she had ALS (amyotropic lateral sclerosis), the same illness that killed Morrie Schwartz. Her doctor said something like, "Evy the results are in and our worst fears have been confirmed. It is ALS, Lou Gerigs' disease. As a nurse, you know that it is a terminal condition. I'm sorry, but because of its rapid progression in your case, I'm afraid that you probably only have about six months to live. I'm sorry." And he turned and left the room without ever once looking at Evy.

Evy was in shock, six months to live, SIX MONTHS TO LIVE! Evy decided to make a time line of her life. She wanted to figure how she got where she was so that the next six months she could do something new. She wanted to make those last six months the best six months.

She decided to examine her development over the breadth of her life. In making her time line she looked at four different dimensions: physical, mental, emotional, and spiritual. Physically, she was overweight and had contractures of an upper and lower extremity secondary to polio as a child. She had been in an iron lung as part of her therapy, but was cute as a button so she was chosen as a polio poster child. Those were the results of her physical exam.

Mentally, she was a powerhouse. This came about as a result of her rebellion against her third grade teacher. She became a star student as a result. Her teacher told Evy that she didn't need to learn her academic lessons because with her handicap she would always be taken care of. She was told she didn't need to keep up with the rest of the class. According to her teacher, Evy should have been placed in the Omaha school for the handicapped, not in her class. This teacher also told Evy's classmates not to play with her since they might catch her polio. So, Evy decided right then that she would prove her teacher wrong. Having had her feelings of inadequacy reinforced by her teacher did not keep Evy down. In fact, it provided energy to validate her right to be in that class. She learned her lessons better than anyone else. She became the best student in her class, won spelling bees, oratory contests and continued to outperform her classmates throughout school. She graduated as the valedictorian of her high school class and went off to a successful college career. She continued her excellent performance throughout nursing school and went on to receive a master's degree. Mentally, she was a peak performer.

Emotionally, however, she was the inverse. As she looked over her life she saw a great deal of depression. In spite of her academic brilliance she did not feel like a star. She was really good at what she did in the field of action. On a competitive basis she was on top. But, she saw herself on the bottom. She was so depressed in high school that she drove her car off the road hoping to hit a tree and never wake up. She missed the tree. Her mental superiority was not enough to compensate for her emotional inferiority and more often than not, she was depressed.

What about her spiritual life? To Evy, spirituality was always synonymous with service. As she examined her life she saw a huge commitment to service. But all of that service was what she described as type one or type two service. Type one service was what she called R&R service. It was service done for reward or recognition. When Evy was a child she had been a candy striper at a local hospital. Evy went to the volunteer leadership and inquired as to the most number of hours that anyone had ever candy striped in a year. She smashed the record and received recognition for her efforts and a plaque was placed on the hospital wall. That was type one service, service done for reward or recognition.

Type two service was service done out of a sense of duty. "On my honor I promise to do my best, to do my duty to God and my country and to obey the scout law. To help other people at all times . . ." Does this sound familiar? Boy and girl scouts memorize their respective scout oaths as part of their training. Evy did her duty by going into nursing so she could "help other people at all times." She accomplished this by landing a job in the intensive care unit. Here she learned to give intensive care to her patients.

Now we come back to the why question. Evy's whole life she had been involved in service. Why? Perhaps that type one service done for reward or recognition is psychic compensation for feelings of inadequacy. If people can get high enough marks from others for their efforts on behalf of the suffering masses, doesn't that prove their worth? Service done out of a sense of duty, type two service, is a concrete way to demonstrate that people are adequate to take their place with the other grownups and do their part as responsible citizens in the community. The military is all about that kind of service. In fact, that is why they call it military service. This is so prominent in the collective consciousness of the culture that if people were to ask someone if they were in "the service," their first response would be with reference to the military. Military service is about giving time, effort, energy, and perhaps life as people defend their country. It's about using force to defeat an enemy. It's about using power to kill. That is not lamb power. That is not love power. That is not spiritual. Martin Luther King, Jr. would most likely agree.

Evy knew that she wanted to be involved in service for her last six months. But it would have to be a different kind of service. She saw that her previous life of service had been about "doing for others." She wanted to be involved with others but in a different, new way. She wanted to serve, but it would have to be what she called type three service. Type three service would have something to do with love and acceptance.

Evy had a problem, however. She discovered that she was the problem because she couldn't love and accept herself. To conquer this, she did an exercise each day in which she looked at herself naked in the mirror. She would look at the person looking back at her in the mirror and write down her thoughts. What came up as she gazed in the glass was negative. She wrote every negative thought but persevered until she finally was able to see something positive about the person looking back. It might have been her hands as they were not affected by the polio.

In the process of breaking through all of that negativity to find something positive to write down, something changed. She found other positive things to note in her book and eventually was able to do what had eluded her. She began to accept the woman in the mirror. And she began to love her.

Then she took that love and acceptance and gave it away. She gave it away to everyone she met. Indiscriminately she poured her love and acceptance into anyone who came into the flashlight of her attention. Her energy flowed easily out to others; not to heal them, not to make them feel better, not because it was her duty, not for what she would get back from them, not to please them, but because of how good she felt serving. She was doing what she was doing because she only had a short amount of time to live and she wanted to make that time the best time of her life. She was giving away what she needed. And in the process of the outflow, in the act of giving, she was filled. She went to the well. As she emptied her bucket of love and acceptance into the people she served she was simultaneously replenished. This type three service served her.

Because she was acting out of her own center, doing what she wanted to do to meet her own needs, there was no reason to be ego inflated behind her service. She wasn't doing it for others. She was doing it for herself. She was actually being selfish because she was doing what made *her* feel better. Miraculously, she did feel better. She had a great six months, then another six, and another . . . Evy Macdonald was one of the first people in the world to be cured of ALS. She did what she did not to make her disease go away. She did what she did to make the most out of the short time she had to live. If she were only to have six more months she wanted them to be the best six.

Later, Evy's neurologist invited Evy to be on a panel at a medical meeting in Italy with neurologists from 27 countries. She had a chance to talk about her healing. By extending the invitation, her neurologist had a chance to learn more from Evy. Why didn't he look at Evy when he told her she had six months to live? Perhaps it had something to do with the risk involved of getting emotionally involved. He might cry. Maybe he was feeling inadequate because he couldn't "fix" Evy's problem. Regardless of the doctor's reason, Evy was denied the comfort of his gaze and his full presence at a time when she really needed his warmth, his love, and acceptance. Perhaps type three service should be taught in medical school since medicine *is* a service profession.

■ THE IMPACT OF EVY'S STORY

I first heard Evy's remarkable story at a two day board retreat of the American Holistic Medical Association. I was very impressed with Evy and her story. And I have continued to be impressed over the years. Evy published an article about the care of patients and family members affected by ALS. The article was excellent, but what really struck me was the fact that nowhere did it mention that the author was afflicted with the disease.

The second example has to do with how Evy has chosen to live her life. She became a member of the New Roadmap Foundation in Seattle. This group of servants lives in a community and has a membership that is unique in my experience. Each member of the community has figured out how to live their lives without needing to work for money. They have learned to live on what they have saved or invested so that any labor that they choose to do does not require financial compensation. Many members use the approach to money that Joe Domingues and Vicki Robin wrote about in their book *Your Money or Your Life.*[3] They save money by living communally and sharing expenses. Therefore, they need less. They have discovered something most of us have never learned, what is enough. They have enough so they do not need more.

They live lives of service, doing only what they want to do or what they are called to do. Money is not the driver of the decision making process. They have it in perspective. So, having a healthy, though not normal relationship with money, they are free to serve as they choose. If you want to have Evy come speak at a meeting you'll just need to cover her expenses. She doesn't need your money. She has enough. That's impressive.

Loaves of Bread and A Few Fish

Evy's story is a new version of a very ancient tale. There's a story of this man who was a great raconteur and after speaking to a large gathering, the attendees were hungry. There were no concessions there to offer food for sale. But, there were a couple of people there with a few loaves of bread, and a few fish. The speaker suggested that the holders of the fish and bread distribute their food to feed the assembled masses. There was some hesitancy by those with the food as there was little food and many people. Any fool could see that the people far outnumbered the food and there could be problems if a few got food, but most had none. The speaker said to trust him on this one and give what they had away. As their hands reached in to grab and pass out the bread and fish their stocks were instantly replenished. The faster they doled it out the faster it was replaced. In this way, the people were fed. To serve those assembled they had to take action. For until they acted no one was fed. But they had to trust that the speaker knew what he was talking about. This story is about food—not the bread and fish—but the food that nourishes the soul.

What we have through type three service is a psychology of abundance. Both the speaker and Evy's perspective is that people always have what they need and it is just enough for whoever shows up, so give it away. The economics of the speaker and Evy is spiritual in which love is the unit of exchange and the more people give it away the more they have of it. Evy was sick and needed healing. The speaker was a healer and needed patients. Evy got what she needed. So did the speaker. Through her illness Evy came to a gnosis, a knowing that was not a part of her acculturation, even the culture of her own healing profession. Through her illness and subsequent gnosis, Evy came to an epignosis, an understanding that allowed her to better serve her culture, including the culture of the whole of the healing profession.

And the speaker? His healing work got him into trouble with the holders of the cultural flame. They put heat on him, made it hot for him, to no avail. For he was burning already with the love that is the creative impulse of the manifest and unmanifest worlds. He burned with the mystery that is the paradox without name.

> Who then devised the torment? Love.
> Love is the unfamiliar Name
> Behind the hands that wove
> The intolerable shirt of flame

Which human power cannot remove.
We only live, only surprise
Consumed by either fire or fire.

T.S. Eliot, Little Gidding, IV

What clinicians are asked to risk as they serve pales in comparison to the work the speaker was called to do. Evy got her disease and healed her life. In so doing she showed people how to heal theirs. The speaker had his health and gave his life. In so doing, he showed people how to find theirs. "I once was lost." But both of them were/are servants and the finding and the healing involved giving love and acceptance. Those two are more precious than life. Share the wealth and serve themselves. And their burning will light the way. That's service.

And the lives of Evy and the speaker also demonstrate how all the rest of the spiritual principles are integrated in the way people serve and the why of that service. Evy was honest, honestly accepting the actual reality of her disease. She had hope, hoping that there was some meaning to be derived, something to know from her illness. She had faith that love and acceptance was important enough to look for with perseverance. Mercy, Mercy, Mercy. She had the guts to face her negative feelings about herself and the courage to then do what had heart, meaning and passion for herself. Evy acted with integrity as she was transparent, congruent. What was going on inside her was revealed outside. She showed a willingness to take action in the world despite her terminal diagnosis. She took on the responsibility of making a difficult situation better, as in "best six months."

She was humble enough to recognize that she needed to change. And after she changed she did not even mention that she had ALS in the article she published on that degenerative disease. She participates in a supportive community so that something larger than herself has the people power to touch her and vice versa. Giving everyone love and acceptance means that Evy would live a life of compassion. For some, perhaps most, of the people she encounters are suffering. And when love touches the suffering of another that is compassion. She has awareness of the vertical yet functions in both worlds. She is awake. Everyday is a present, a gift she was told she would never have.

And what of the speaker? His life has long been an example for the healing community and the world at large. There are others, older ones and not so old. But, here, one old, a healer and one new, a patient will suffice. But they all say the same thing to others. Whatever they have done, so too others can do.

Ways in which you might use service in your practice and encourage your chronically ill patients to do the same:

- There are three types of service. Type 3 service has to do with love and acceptance. Encourage your patients to try this kind of service and be prepared to reap all the benefits from it. This type of service can start at home. It can be with your own spouse or child.
- The benefit of true service is that you don't need or expect anything back.
- Recognize the benefit you receive from the service you give. You should be doing service work because you want to serve. We benefit from serving. There is no shortage of suffering people, no shortage of opportunity to serve.

REFERENCES

1. S. Mitchell, *Tao Te Ching, a New English Version*, Harper Collins, New York, 1992, p. 17.
2. G.E. Vaillant, *The Wisdom of the Ego*, Harvard University Press, 1993, p. 134.
3. Joe Domingues and Vicki Robin, *Your Money or Your Life*, Penguin Books, 1992.

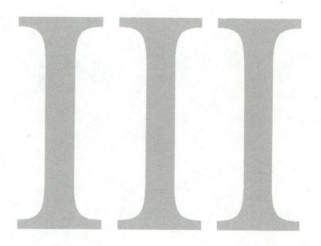

Part III

Conclusion

16

Chapter Sixteen

From Study to Action

John A. Mac Dougall

> On action alone be thy interest, never on its fruits. Let not the
> fruits of action be thy motive, nor be they attachment to inac-
> tion.
>
> *Bhagavad Gita*, 2:27

Thank you for reading this book. All authors want to have their
works read and we do, too. We appreciate the time you have
spent with us. Now we are hoping you will go a step beyond reading
and learning, to action. Having invested time in what we have to
say, we now encourage you to invest time and effort in your own
spiritual growth.

Remember that spirituality consists of the quality or nature of
our relationships in three dimensions: with a Higher Power, with
ourselves, and with other people. Each of the spiritual principles
can be applied in ways that improve our relationships in each of
these three dimensions.

Our suggested method is to pick one spiritual principle that
you would like to enhance in your life: honesty, faith, integrity, service, or any of the twelve. Then pick one dimension of your relationships that you would like to improve: relationships with your
Higher Power, how you feel about yourself or how you regard yourself, or spiritual principle to the chosen dimension of life, choose
one behavior change that you will make, in order to make this possible. Change your behavior, then allow time to evaluate the
results. You may want to give your new behavior time and repeti-

tion, in order to give it a chance to result in a spiritual benefit. If your evaluation is positive, you may want to pick another behavior change, that could advance this spiritual principle in another aspect of life.

For one example, a physician might pick honesty as the principle to be advanced. Relationships with others might be the dimension for action. One behavior change might be to stop signing "gag clauses" in managed care contracts, in which you promise not to discuss anything they don't pay for. A physician with such a problem could assess the results after a year or so. There might be fewer patients and less income. There might be improved relationships with patients and an increased satisfaction with the practice of medicine. Then the physician could evaluate whether the improved relationships were worth the loss of income.

Positive changes in one dimension are likely to spill over into the two dimensions. In this example, giving up "gag clauses," there would be a likely improvement in interpersonal relationships. However, the physician might also feel better about himself or herself, and closer to a Higher Power because of acting according to their spiritual principles.

This is a big project. Even if we made only one behavior change on each principle in each dimension, that's 36 behavior changes. Chances are, we'd want to do many more. Even the first changed behavior will represent spiritual progress.

You may want to make an outline to keep track of our spiritual progress. Here's one format for a weekly self-assessment:

This week, I have been honest, as evidenced by . . .

This week, I have hope, as evidenced by . . .

This week, I have faith in a Higher Power, and in the process of spiritual growth, as evidenced by . . .

This week, I have acted with courage, as evidenced by . . .

This week, I have had integrity, as evidenced by . . .

This week, I have been willing to change, as evidenced by . . .

This week, I have had humility, as evidenced by . . .

This week, I have acted with compassion, as evidenced by . . .

This week, I have been just, as evidenced by . . .

This week, I have persevered in spiritual growth, as evidenced by . . .

This week, I have been spiritually aware, as evidenced by . . .

This week, I have served others, as evidenced by . . .

As we change one behavior at a time, to advance these principles, our weekly report to ourselves will improve. Our attitude and outlook on life will change, and we will enjoy living.

We also invite you to start a dialogue with us. How are you using these spiritual principles in your life? What impact are they having on your life, your work, your play, and your relationships? Your experiences will help us, and we can all benefit together. You are welcome to write us in care of:

Hazelden Information and Education Services
PO Box 176
Center City, MN 55012

Index

3

ISBN 0-07-134717-8

90000

9 780071 347174

WHITE/SPIRITUALITY